OPTIMUM BRAIN POWER

A TOTAL PROGRAM FOR INCREASING YOUR INTELLIGENCE

Miriam Ehrenberg Ph.D.
Otto Ehrenberg Ph.D.

DODD, MEAD & COMPANY
New York

This book was written with the
assistance of Erica Ehrenberg.

A GAMUT BOOK

Copyright © 1985 by Miriam Ehrenberg and Otto Ehrenberg

Published by Dodd, Mead & Company, Inc.
71 Fifth Avenue, New York, N.Y. 10003
Distributed in Canada by
McClelland and Stewart Limited, Toronto
Manufactured in the United States of America
2 3 4 5 6 7 8 9 10

Library of Congress Cataloging in Publication Data

Ehrenberg, Miriam.
   Optimum brain power.

   Includes index.
   1. Intellect.   2. Success.   I. Ehrenberg, Otto.
II. Title.
BF431.E47   1984   153   83-2543
ISBN 0-396-08391-9
ISBN 0-396-09071-0 {PBK}

CONTENTS

To Edith Webster Wax

INTELLIGENCE: WHAT IT IS AND HOW IT GROWS

Although this is the age of self-improvement, of learning how to live better longer, how to say "no" without feeling guilty, how to make love to a man (or a woman), and how to eat well and stay fit, very few of us ever consider the possibility of learning how to become more intelligent. We have accepted the myths about intelligence handed down to us by scientists who have led us to believe that intelligence is an inherited entity that is fixed at birth, like the color of our eyes or the number of our toes. It is assumed that either you have a good brain or you don't. This is just not so. Intelligence is not something you have, but *a way of being that you develop.* It is functioning productively by utilizing your optimum brain potential. Most people are not as intelligent as they could be, not because of their genetic inheritance, but because they use only a fraction of their intellectual capacities. To be able to use those capacities you must first free yourself from the artificial constraints put on your intelligence by the scientific mythmakers. Once you realize the possibilities for increasing your intelligence, you will find that your intelligence is your most undeveloped resource.

MYTHS ABOUT INTELLIGENCE

Society has always been characterized by social distinctions between classes and also by rationalizations to justify the resulting inequities. The most widespread belief, called biological determinism, holds that differences in social class reflect differences in biology. Since some are born better equipped than others, the argument goes, they naturally deserve and get more. In previous eras it was felt that the strong were entitled to a bigger share on the basis of their inherited brawn; in our era it is felt that the intelligent are more deserving on the basis of their inherited brains.

The nineteenth-century scientists who first promulgated the theory of genetic intelligence recognized the need for objective data to corroborate this point of view. They therefore conducted many research studies, and developed many tools to measure intelligence. Although their work had the aura of scientific objectivity, their studies were riddled with errors, ambiguities, and downright distortions of data. Their "pseudoscience," as Jeffrey Blum has called it, nevertheless continued to hold sway. Many scientists today, as well as the lay public, still believe in the truth of genetically determined differences in intelligence. The following short review of the faulty research conducted by the scientific myth makers should help to dispel this belief. Readers interested in a more detailed exploration may want to read Jeffrey Blum's *Pseudoscience and Mental Ability* as well as Steven Jay Gould's *The Mismeasure of Man.*

Among the earliest inquiries into genetic differences in intelligence were those conducted by an American physician and scientist, Samuel George Morton, who sought to prove that the different races derived their different statuses in life from their inherited biological differences, most notably brain size. He collected skulls of different races and measured the cranial cavity, which provides a fairly accurate measure of the brain it once held. Morton's data were published in the mid-1800s and showed whites having the biggest brain, followed by Indians and blacks, with the biggest white brains belonging to Anglo-Saxons, followed by Jews and then Hindus, thus seemingly proving that social status resulted from innate cranial capacity. As biologist Steven Jay Gould has demonstrated, however, Morton used incorrect mathematical procedures in averaging his data, ignored some data completely, and did not control for body size. Reanalyzing the data, Gould found that the supposed race differences in brain size disappeared once differences in body stature of the specimens used were controlled. Apparently no one in Morton's time bothered to check his data because his findings were in line with the social prejudices of the day.

Brain measurement, or craniometry, was carried on in Europe by other eminent scientists, including Paul Broca. The European studies, too, were riddled with poor controls and manipulation of data to accord with the beliefs of the investigators. By and large these studies were said to prove the notion that lower class members, people of dark skin color, and women were of small brain size and inferior intelligence. When data were unearthed that contradicted this theory, such as the finding that eminent white men who were university professors had small brains, circular reasoning was employed to allow the theory to stand intact. It was decided that these men were really not so smart after all, witness their small brain size.

Craniometry gave way to a more modern instrument—that of the intelligence test—which is imputed to measure intelligence more accurately than brain size. The field of intelligence testing, unfortunately, shows as much, if not more, distortion of data, circularity of argument, and misinterpretation of fact as the field of craniometry does. The chapter "Raising Your IQ" covers some of the problems in the way IQ tests are constructed. What follows is a brief review of some of the faulty and misleading thinking that went into their creation.

The first person to have attempted testing intelligence directly was Francis Galton, a Victorian gentleman, scholar, and cousin of Charles Darwin. He believed that social inequalities were reflections of differences in inherited mental capacities, and set out to prove that persons of eminence were more intelligent than others, occupying their exalted positions by virtue of their superior intellectual inheritance. In his first attempt to test intelligence he measured sensory acuity and speed of motor reaction, but he found that the differences obtained did not discriminate between those of high and low status. In another attempt to prove his theory, Galton studied the lineage of famous people and, finding that eminence clustered in families, took that as evidence that talent is hereditary. He not only incorrectly equated eminence with intelligence, but overlooked that the clustering could be a by-product of shared superior opportunity rather than a result of shared superior endowment. Galton, in fact, denied the role of environmental influences on intelligence. After conducting other studies to verify the relationship between inherited intelligence and social differences, Galton became a spokesman for the eugenics movement, which advocated controlling the birth rate of the lower, and presumably less intelligent, classes.

Galton had tried, but failed, to develop a method of measuring intelligence. What the biological determinists needed was an instrument that could provide a numerical rank or score of intellectual capability, and the IQ test thus came into being.

e testing had the appearance of scientific accuracy but
IQ tests were designed in such ways that certain
ld do well and others not. When persons of high
and high status performed well as predicted while those
of low status scored low, it was induced, by circular logic, that
the tests were a valid measure of intelligence, because the high-
status groups were "obviously" more intelligent. The data that
the testmakers offered to prove either the validity of their tests or
the concept of genetic intelligence were often without substance
and, in many cases, consciously manipulated to serve their ends.
Henry Goddard, for instance, the first popularizer of IQ testing
in America, claimed to have proven that low status was a result
of inherited low mental capacity. In an early study conducted in
1912, he and his associate rated the facial expressions of a community of poor farmers, and decided the faces all indicated
arrested mental development, thereby "proving" that peasants
were held in low condition by their feeblemindedness. It was
only in 1980 that research revealed that some of the photos were
touched up by Goddard to provide a "dull" and feebleminded
look.

Lewis Terman, whose Stanford-Binet is probably the best
known intelligence test in the country, also contributed research
findings to "prove" the innateness of intelligence. He gave his
IQ test to members of various occupational groups and concluded that those holding higher-status positions did so by virtue of their greater innate intelligence, as evidenced by their
higher IQ scores. When occupational groups of low status
achieved a high IQ, he dismissed these results, claiming that
such persons must have lacked other desirable innate qualities
that kept them from rising higher on the prestige ladder. Terman and his associates also conducted the *Genetic Studies of
Genius*, published in the 1920s, to demonstrate how high IQ is
inherited by eminent personages. The methodology was as follows: after reading published biographic information on historically eminent people, an IQ score was estimated for each by
adding extra points to a base of 100 for each accomplishment,
and subtracting points for "unintelligent" traits such as rebel-
liousness. The assignment of an IQ score for each of these dead
eminences gave the study the aura of scientific objectivity. However, not all the raters agreed on the IQ that was assigned and the
ratings of those who disagreed too markedly were thrown out,
thereby eliminating almost half the "data." A more glaring

problem was the fact that the IQ ratings reflected the amount of published data on the subjects rather than their actual performance. Thus Copernicus, who left behind little data on his early years, could not receive many IQ points, and ended up with an IQ score of only 105, compared to Francis Galton, who left copious notes on his activities in childhood and adulthood and ended up with an IQ of 200. This despite the fact that Copernicus left us with a new conception of the universe, while Galton left us with an erroneous idea about the nature of intelligence!

Other later attempts to prove that intelligence was transmitted by the genes and that environment played a minimal role were focused on studies comparing IQ score differences between pairs of identical twins raised in different homes with those of identical twins raised in the same home, and with nongenetically related children raised in the same home. The findings of these studies, conducted over several decades, were generally reported to show that IQ correlated about 80 percent with heredity and 20 percent with environment. Scientific analyses of the heritability studies put the credibility of these figures into great doubt. Leon Kamin's analysis in *The Science and Politics of IQ* concluded that they are meaningless, being based on inadequate research studies, misinterpretation of data, and even deception. Evidence has also been uncovered that two major English researchers, Karl Pearson and Cyril Burt, who presented some of the strongest evidence of genetic determination, distorted data of studies they supervised to show higher degrees of heritability. Cyril Burt even went so far as to fabricate the data he needed to support his point of view. In light of the unsound data, all that can be said on the basis of the heritability studies is that there is no valid evidence on which to conclude that intelligence is a fixed, genetically transmitted characteristic.

THE TRUTHS ABOUT INTELLIGENCE

The myths about intelligence stem from the common fallacy of "reification"—turning an abstract concept into a real thing. Because we have a word called "intelligence" it is assumed that there is a concrete entity corresponding to that name, located in our heads. Intelligence, however, like many other human attributes, is not something tangible that can be seen, located, or measured. Rather, it manifests itself in the way we behave and relate to the world. It is a quality of being that we develop and that is shaped by our experiences.

We are all born with the capacity for intelligent behavior, barring, of course, some kind of damage to our systems. Nobody inherits a specific quantity of intelligence. Whether or not we will use our intellectual potential depends primarily on the life experiences we encounter and make for ourselves. An analogy with our other capacities makes this clearer. We are all born with the potential for locomotion, again barring physical damage. We all learn to walk, because this requires relatively little effort and very little in the way of environmental supports. We don't, however, all learn to swim, and particularly to swim well. If you live in a town where there is no lake or pool, you are not going to be able to learn how to swim. Similarly, if you do live near water but have to spend all your spare time working, you will not have time to learn how to swim. Or, if you are undernourished and weak and therefore lack coordination, you will not learn how to swim. At the other extreme, if you are healthy, have a pool in your backyard, and your mother is a swimming coach or hires one to train you, you may end up winning an Olympic medal. These differences in swimming ability do not mean that some people have higher SQs, or Swimming Quotients, than others or that they inherited more swimming ability. All it shows is that if you have the opportunity and training you will become a better swimmer.

The same holds true for intelligence. If left alone, you will use and develop some of your intellectual potential, but if you are in an enriched environment that provides lots of stimulation, training, and opportunity, your intelligence will soar. The major impediment to greater intelligence is not insufficient innate capacities, but insufficient use of capacities we already possess.

Research on the brain reveals it has biological complexity of staggering dimensions, estimated up to 100 billion neurons, 10 billion in the cortex alone, and each neuron connected to hundreds of others by anywhere from 100 to 10,000 synaptic junctions. The total number of interconnections in the brain is in the order of trillions. Nothing we have made, even the most intricate computers, begins to approach the complexity of the brain. Yet, only a small part of this potential is ever used. It is estimated that less than 10 percent of the nerve cells and their possible connections are developed in an average adult brain.

Obviously there is a tremendous reserve of brain power going to waste. In view of this large reserve, it is reasonable to assume that differences in intelligence relate more to the extent to which this potential is developed than to the quantity of brain cells with which one is born.

Maintaining the physical health of the brain is one factor influencing the development of intelligence. Inadequate diet or the presence of toxins interferes with the growth of a healthy nervous system and brain. When the brains of children who died of malnutrition in the first year of life were compared to those of normal children who died through accidental causes, it was found that the former had fewer brain cells and an overall decrease in brain size. The brain differences also show up in behavior. Studies of children suffering from malnutrition show marked decreases in their behavioral performance; children provided with adequate diets show significantly more activity, energy, curiosity, and playfulness. The importance of nutrition, however, does not stop in infancy but continues throughout life. Recent findings indicate that adult brains too are significantly influenced by diet.

Providing adequate stimulation is another essential ingredient of intellectual growth. Research studies of gifted persons show that most were exposed to exceptionally high levels of intellectual stimulation in childhood and were brought up in active environments by parents who devoted themselves to the children's education, which typically began well before school age.

Research similarly indicates that a lack of stimulation retards mental development. Many studies have shown that children who grow up in sterile environments, whether stemming from neglect or intellectual impoverishment, develop subnormal intelligence. Children reared in institutional settings that provided little opportunity for interaction with others, grew up with serious mental deficiencies. The higher than average rate of mental retardation among children born prematurely and isolated in incubators has recently been shown to be a consequence of insufficient stimulation after birth rather than a result of incomplete gestation.

The effects of stimulation in developing intelligence are not only observable on a behavioral level but on a physical level as well. A stimulating environment provokes the individual to activity, thereby exercising the brain and helping to establish neural circuits that create permanent changes in the physical structure of the brain. For example, when rat litters were separated into two groups and one placed in a sterile environment and the other in an enriched environment, it did not take long for differences in the size and chemical composition of their brain cells to occur. The brains of mature animals also responded to an enriched environment, though these changes took longer to achieve.

Still one other factor has an important impact on the development of intelligence: attitude. In order for intelligence to grow, there first has to be the expectation of growth. Research indicates that parental encouragement and an attitude of high expectation is vital in the development of intellectual potential. Persons who are encouraged to be independent, to think, to question, and to explore, develop into more intelligent beings than those who are kept dependent and punished for innovative thought and queries.

DEFINING INTELLIGENCE

So far we have talked about how intelligence develops but have not really discussed what comprises it. Historically, psychologists have had difficulty defining just what intelligence is. Their definitions have centered on the ability to think abstractly and to solve problems. They see intelligence as primarily composed of academic-type skills—essentially the same type of skills that are measured by intelligence tests. Indeed, because of the uncertainty about what intelligence is, one definition used by psychologists is that intelligence is what is measured by intelligence tests!

Despite psychologists' difficulty with defining intelligence, the public seems to know what it means. A recent study conducted by Robert Sternberg, a psychologist at Yale, revealed that people by and large agree on what intelligence is and are adept at making quick assessments of another's intelligence level. Lay people have a broader view of intelligence than the experts, placing emphasis on what Sternberg calls the "social-cultural" aspects of intelligence. To be intelligent in the psychology laboratory means having a good vocabulary, reading with high comprehension, posing problems in an optimal way, and making good decisions; but to be intelligent in the world at large means all that plus admitting mistakes, having a social conscience, thinking before doing, being interested in the world, having sensitivity to other people's needs, and being honest with oneself and others.

One reason that psychologists have a narrower view of intelligence is that they tend to value those intellectual skills that are necessary to their scientific pursuits, such as the ability to analyze data and follow logical thought sequences, and to undervalue skills that are less immediately applicable, such as sensitivity and intuition. At the extreme, some psychologists believe that the so-called artificial intelligence of computers, with its enormous data-handling possibilities, can actually surpass human intelligence. However, while it is already possible for a computer to beat a grand master at a game of chess, it is inconceivable that a computer (which cannot be programmed to be sensitive to nuances) could ever beat a master at a game of poker.

Recent research has validated the existence of mental capacities that even go beyond those included in the broad lay definition of intelligent behavior. Biofeedback techniques, as well as meditation techniques, have demonstrated how bodily processes assumed to be involuntary, such as blood pressure and pulse rate, can be controlled by the mind that is trained. Similarly, recent research in the Soviet Union and the United States has demonstrated that people can also use their minds to communicate telepathically and to move objects through space. Extrasensory perception appears now not to be "extra" at all but to refer to a normal part of the sensorium that most people just don't use, or even know exists.

It is difficult to offer a definition of intelligence because it is not an entity but an evolving process. We all know more or less what we can do at this moment, but we have no idea what we are capable of doing once we take off the self-imposed lids. It is only when we begin to accept the extraordinary powers of our minds that we can free our minds to realize them. You can be more intelligent, and only by exercising that capacity will you come to know more fully what intelligence is.

DEVELOPING YOUR INTELLIGENCE

The idea of improving intelligence is not new, although it has never really taken hold. Some have tried in the past to arouse interest in the idea of teaching people to be more intelligent, but have not met with much enthusiasm. One of the early pioneers in this field was a nineteenth-century Austrian clergyman named Karl Witte. He developed a method for training children to have superior intellects, but his work fell into obscurity and the children reared according to his methods were isolated cases rather than the rule. Others were able to attract more attention to their work. Maria Montessori, the first Italian woman doctor, earned an international reputation by developing early learning techniques for children. She discovered that optimal learning took place at lower ages than was commonly believed; for instance, that it is easier for a child to learn to read and write around four years of age than six, the normal age for starting school. Montessori became convinced through her work that traditional education does not tap the true capacities of children and thereby produces people who function below their natural potential. Montessori schools opened in many parts of the world, but they did not make much headway in the United States, partially because educational psychologists thought that accelerated learning interfered with children's emotional adjustment, another idea bred by science that has been proven wrong. A few other pioneers in the movement to develop the intelligence of children and students should be mentioned: Siegfried and Theresa Engelmann, who present their method in *Give Your Child a Superior Mind*; and Arthur Whimbey, whose ideas are contained in *Intelligence Can Be Taught*.

More recently, there have been attempts to improve the thinking capacity of adults as well as of children. Courses in problem-solving have been offered by various colleges including UCLA, Carnegie Mellon Institute, and the University of Massachusetts, and by private institutes such as those run by Edward de Bono. In the same vein, the government of Venezuela has initiated a Ministry of State for the Development of Human Intelligence, dedicated to expanding the thinking capacity of its citizens.

These programs represent an exciting change from previous notions about intelligence in their recognition of the fluid nature of intelligence and the possibilities for its growth. They do not, however, go far enough, maintaining the focus on academic-type skills, which represent only a part of our intelligence. In this book we will show you how to increase your intelligence on all levels.

Several basic principles underlie the material and exercises presented in this book. First, you have to know what resources you have and then you have to learn how to use them. Let's take a camera as an analogy. A good camera comes equipped with a variable lens opening, an adjustable shutter speed, and probably telephoto and wide-angle lenses. To make use of the capabilities of this camera, you have to understand what these features are and know how they work. If you want to take really good pictures, you also have to know what is worth shooting and what film to feed your camera to provide the results you want. Your brain, like a camera, comes equipped with many special features. If you know how it works, the results can be terrific. As with a camera, you can learn how to focus on detail or widen your field of vision; you can learn how to get more varied impressions and develop memory prints that will not fade; you can learn to differentiate between what is worth imprinting on your mind and what will make for a meaningless print that will just clutter up your memory scrapbook. Reading this book and practicing working with your brain will enable you to use your latent talents. Each chapter covers a different aspect of intelligence, including how the process works and exercises for developing that particular facet of your intellect. You do not necessarily have to read the chapters in order; you can start with those that are most interesting to you. We do, however, urge you eventually to study them all, because the various aspects discussed are integral parts of your intelligence and reinforce one another.

We also suggest that you do all the exercises in this book, even the ones involving functions that you are not concerned about. If you concentrate on just some aspects of intellectual activity and ignore the others, you leave parts of your brain idle. The more of your brain that you use and the more you keep all the cells and circuitry activated, the healthier your entire brain will be. Bicycling, for example, may be particularly good for developing your leg muscles, but it tones up your whole body in the process —you are forced to breathe more deeply, coordinate your eye and hand movements to go along with your pedaling, and so forth. The same principle applies to the brain—if you exercise one part, you exercise it all.

Ultimately, improving your intelligence will depend on the attitude you take to your own possibilities. There is a direct relationship between your expectations and what you can do, as discussed in the chapter "Emotions and Intelligence." You must become convinced of the manifold possibilities you have waiting to be developed. The key to greater intelligence is understanding what your mind can do, giving yourself lots of exercise in doing it, and having the faith in your own capacities of achievement.

PROCESSING VERBAL INFORMATION

The use of language constitutes the essential difference between humans and animals. Our ability to name things gives us power over them in that we can then manipulate them symbolically. This almost magical power of words is recognized in folklore as well as in religion. Rumpelstiltskin, for instance, loses his power when his name is discovered. God not only commands that the name of the Lord not be taken in vain, but creates order out of chaos through the word. The importance of language to us as individuals was vividly expressed by Helen Keller when she described the moment she first understood what a word was: "Suddenly I felt a misty consciousness . . . I knew then that w-a-t-e-r meant the wonderful cool something that was flowing over my hand. That living word awakened my soul, and . . . set it free. . . . Everything had a name, and each name gave birth to a new thought . . . every object which I touched seemed to quicken with life. That was because I saw everything with the strange new sight that had come to me."

Words, and their endless combinations into statements, ideas, and concepts, provide us with the basic units of thought. Most of the information transmitted to us comes via the use of language and most of our thought occurs by means of linguistic signs. Other avenues of information are also available to us and we learn a lot about the world through our senses, but language plays a major role in helping us order and understand what we take in through these channels. Without a conceptual framework with which to interpret sensory material, it would not be meaningful to us. Similarly, much of the information to which we are exposed, such as numerical data, formulas, or charts, becomes intelligible to us only in the context of verbal concepts. We are not concerned purely with numbers but with what they are telling us about a particular situation. Certainly then, the ability to acquire and process verbal information is fundamental to building intelligence.

ACQUIRING INFORMATION

The more verbal information you acquire, the more intelligent you can be. Stored information not only allows you to deal intelligently with the world on the basis of that knowledge, but also enables you to understand better the new information that comes in. If you know arithmetic, you are better able to take in algebra. If you know English grammar, you are better able to learn French grammar. If you know the facts of Latin American history, you can better understand the present conflict in El Salvador.

Acquiring information builds neural pathways that expand your brain's capacity. The more you take in now, the more you will be able to take in later. Did you ever notice how a dry sponge does not mop up moisture well? Or how dried up soil cannot absorb the rain, which then just runs off the surface? Well, an arid mind is the same. One of the most important principles in being more intelligent is to drink up as much information as you can.

Despite the "information explosion," very few people expose themselves to even a tiny fraction of what they could absorb. Let's take you. Do you read the newspaper every day? Do you go through the whole paper or just read the sections you are interested in? Could you give a quick synopsis of all the items covered in today's paper? Most likely you can't, and most likely your attitude has been, "Why fill my head with a lot of stuff that doesn't interest me?" Of course, you want to pay more attention to your areas of interest, but to build your intelligence you need to broaden your areas of information. You don't have to read all the articles, but you should read all the story headings and perhaps the lead paragraphs so that you are aware of everything that is happening. You will probably find yourself getting interested in new areas and thereby understanding more about your prime areas of interest. Whenever possible, browse through all the written material that comes your way. Two newspapers are better than one because they often cover different items or give you different perspectives on the same events. You can profitably go to the library and browse through the magazine shelf every week. Don't just look through your favorite, but give them all the once-over: find out what is happening where, who is doing what, how things are getting done. Some magazines, like *Time* and *Newsweek*, have sections covering different spheres of life. They provide a good overview of events, but are not sufficient because they tend to fill you in on headline items rather than offbeat and often more important news. The less popular "non-establishment" press is much more likely to alert you to such topics as governmental abuses, helpful vitamins and herbs, alternatives to expensive medical care, the benefits of Swiss bank accounts, and loads of other bits and pieces that you need for intelligent living.

In addition to keeping up with current news and periodicals, it is also a good idea for you to set aside some time for browsing through the library shelves that you ordinarily ignore. Have you ever checked through the art, financial, ecology, literary criticism, or computer sections? Even if at first you do not want to borrow any of these books to read through, make it a habit to review the books on the shelf to give you an overview of what is going on. Check the titles, glance through the chapter headings, leaf through the books, read the dust jackets.

At this point you may well want to ask why it is so important for you to acquaint yourself with information from different fields. The reason is that to understand anything well you have to understand everything well enough to see it in context. In previous times, knowledgeable people used to be generalists— they were well versed in all fields. The typical "Renaissance man" was a person of broad interests and skills. The age of technical development, however, brought with it an emphasis on specialization and generations of persons known as physicists, chemists, biologists, sociologists, economists, botanists, plus others with expertise in narrowly defined fields. It is being rediscovered of late that knowledge cannot be compartmentalized and that narrow specialists cannot even perform well at their specialty without broader-based knowledge. The last twenty years have given birth to new "specialists" who, of necessity, have had to widen their field in order to perform adequately. These persons are known as biochemists, medical sociologists, forensic psychiatrists, psycholinguists, to name but a few. Perhaps nowhere more than in the field of medicine has the danger of narrow specialization made itself felt. Physicians too are starting to become aware of the need for persons trained in treating the whole body rather than its isolated parts and so the field of holistic medicine is now coming into its own. Just as our body is more than a sum of its parts, our world is also more than a sum of its parts, and to understand the world and be intelligent in it we need to have a wide view.

We have stressed so far the importance of enlarging the scope of your reading matter. There are, of course, other sources of verbal information besides the printed page. TV is a popular medium, but despite its popularity, TV has limited usefulness as a source of verbal information. The newscasts provide minimal coverage of events and most of their time is taken up by "anchorpersons" acting cute with each other. The weekly series of situation comedies, soap operas, and dramas all tend to follow the same formula and provide very little usable information. The most valuable programs are the documentaries, some of the theater pieces that have been adapted or filmed for TV, and movie classics. Of course, TV can be fun, and it is perfectly fine to amuse yourself with it. However, it more often tranquilizes rather than stimulates your mind. Unlike reading, which actively engages your mind, and forces your participation, TV viewing catches your attention and does the thinking for you.

TV has a blunting effect on your intelligence in yet another way. By supplying you with a steady stream of ready-made images, it impedes your ability to visualize. Robert Sommer, a professor of psychology and environmental studies, noted: "People are watching more and seeing less." Since visualization is an important aid in memory and thinking, as discussed in other parts of this book, it is apparent that TV is a questionable source of information.

Although our ears are important receptors for verbal information, we usually don't make very good use of them. We have become conditioned by listening to teachers, lecturers, and various electronic devices to take a passive stance toward input from these sources. Passive listening, though, is not much better than TV viewing. Interrupting a speaker to ask questions or discuss a particular point helps you understand the information better. In reading, you set your own pace and create your own pauses to ponder a point. Asking questions and interacting with a lecturer or speaker enables you to obtain the same benefits. The reason that debate has always been recognized as an excellent medium for transmitting ideas and sharpening minds is that it is so intensely engaging. In your everyday verbal encounters, you often have the choice between making them active and informative or dull and less meaningful.

REJECTING INFORMATION

What we take in is limited not only by lack of exposure, but also by our tendency to reject information. We constantly come across information that, for one reason or another, is ignored or rejected by us. This is, of course, very damaging to the development of our intelligence, and being aware of this tendency will help to minimize it. Let's see how and why it works.

Everybody builds up a set of beliefs and attitudes, which helps to orient the way she or he deals with the world. We have beliefs about religion, sex, politics, and taxes, to name only a few, and these beliefs form integrated systems. If you know a person's attitudes about religion, you can predict fairly accurately what that person's views on sex, politics, and taxes are like. Catholics tend to frown at premarital sex or feel guilty about it; Moslems feel justified in stoning those who engage in it. For Zen Buddhists premarital sex is often irrelevant and for Protestants it is generally a matter of individual conscience. Similarly, chances are very high that someone who is anti-abortion is politically conservative, and that someone who is pro-abortion is more to the center or left. Our beliefs form balanced patterns that help us maintain our emotional equilibrium. To preserve our equanimity we try to keep our belief system from being disrupted. What this means, in effect, is that we tend to shut ourselves off from any information that threatens the belief system. When you are exposed to information that is contrary to your beliefs, a process called "cognitive dissonance" sets in. If the dissonance remains, you are going to feel stress. There are only two ways to avoid this stress: either you avoid new information that may create cognitive dissonance, or you modify your belief system to accommodate this new information. Obviously, the way to be more intelligent is to consider new information rather than to close your eyes and ears. If there is a conflict between your ideas and the new information and you let yourself become fully acquainted with the new material, you may find that it is less compelling than you thought and end up with a stronger set of beliefs than before. If, on the other hand, the new information is as compelling as you feared, take heart and modify your old ideas for what will then become a more intelligent set of beliefs.

Not only are there inner barriers to changing our beliefs; this process also is frowned upon by society. "Changing your mind" has a negative connotation that is associated with weakness and typically ascribed to so-called "fickle women." It is assumed that when you "change your mind" you are really letting someone else's mind take over for you, or exchanging another's mind for your own. Actually, when you modify your beliefs, you are not "changing your mind" but using your mind to its fullest. Only an intelligent mind has the flexibility to adapt to new information, to throw out worthless ideas, and the resourcefulness to build up new belief systems that are able to account for a wider variety of facts and experiences. To build your intelligence you have to be open to new ideas.

MISSING OUT ON INFORMATION

Sometimes important information slips by us because we program ourselves not to see it. Unlike the situation that arises when we reject information because we do not want to deal with it, when we miss out on information, we are not even aware of it. The information is usually lost to us because we set our minds on looking for other types of information and thereby narrow our focus to take in only preselected items. Sometimes this can be a valuable device. Suppose you want to learn about the brain. If you pick up a physiology book it makes a great deal of sense to read just the chapters on the brain and the nervous system rather than plodding through the whole book. But such selectivity can also prove limiting. If you wanted to find out about care of your brain, you would have to look at the chapter on the circulatory system to find out how the brain gets fed, and at the chapter on temperature regulation to find out about the danger of fever to the brain, and so on. Often we don't know in advance just what information we want and it is therefore helpful to take a broad scan so that the relevant information becomes apparent. In the example of the physiology book, you can miss out on important information by reading one chapter rather than another. It is also possible to miss out on information contained within the chapter you do read. What happens is that your focus is still limited by what fits into your framework. Let's see how that works.

Exercise

Read the list below, and then answer the questions at the bottom of the following page.

THE SENSES
visual
auditory
olfactory
tactile
kinesthetic

Probably you could not answer the question properly and, of course, if you are reading a chapter on the sense organs it is irrelevant what kind of type the material is printed in, just as long as you understand what the type is saying. This example was merely meant to show you how easy it is to miss out on details that you consider irrelevant. A problem does occur, however, when you make decisions about relevance without sufficient grounds. Let's look at some of those situations.

If you are a murder-mystery fan you are familiar with the wily detectives who can solve all the crimes because they notice some seemingly irrelevant detail that escapes everyone else's attention. Sherlock Holmes, in *Silver Blaze*, for example, is asked:

"Is there any other point to which you would wish to draw my attention?"
"To the curious incident of the dog in the night-time."
"The dog did nothing in the night-time."
"That was the curious incident," remarked Sherlock Holmes.

Arthur Conan Doyle, the creator of Sherlock Holmes, and Edgar Allan Poe, another famed mystery writer, were actually able to apply the principle of noticing the "irrelevant" in real life as well as fiction. Both solved murder cases whose solutions had eluded the police for years. Conan Doyle succeeded by noticing that threatening letters written by the murderer stopped for a period of seven years, a clue ignored by the police. By determining who in the community was away for seven years, Conan Doyle was able to identify the murderer. Similarly, Poe picked up on the fact, published in the newspapers, that the murder victim had disappeared 2½ years before the crime, a clue also ignored by the police. In tracking down the victim's activity at the time of the disappearance, Poe also discovered the murderer. In both these situations, the tendency to close the mind off to material considered irrelevant stopped the police from finding the real killers.

Chances are that you miss noticing relevant information every day. Sometimes it does not matter too much, as in the following situation which we witness almost every time we are in New York City. Some of the bus lines change their scheduled stops during the course of the day. Either they become "limited" and only make express stops, or they change their destination point and go only part of the usual route. It never fails when we get on a "limited" or a short-route bus that some of the passengers get upset because the bus does not stop where they think it should or because they have to dismount and wait for a regular-route bus. The buses are clearly marked, but these people disregard that information. They check to see that they have the right bus line, but not if they have the right bus. Sometimes the consequences of missing out on information can be more serious. Have you ever tried to back off a busy expressway ramp or gone ten miles out of your way to the next exit because you missed a sign? Did you ever have to throw away a shirt or pair of jeans because you did not check the label and learn that it was going to shrink/fade/run?

Not paying attention to as much detail as possible can be costly in more important ways, many of which we come to realize too late. If we fail to notice the fine print in a contract, we are apt to become aware of that only when we have to pay the price. Just as importantly, many opportunities are missed by failing to notice details that can be advantageous to us . . . perhaps an announcement of a low-cost vacation, a job opening, or possibilities of a business deal. Broadening your scope of attention to include more cues will help increase your intelligence and enhance your life.

Closely related to the process of not noticing what we consider irrelevant detail is the tendency to distort such detail to fit in with our preconceptions. Let us see how that works.

Is the list of senses written in capitals, initial capitals, or small print? Is the heading written in capitals, initial capitals, or small print?

Exercise

Below are several familiar phrases. Read each phrase to yourself and after you have read all three write a critical statement about each phrase.

Time and tide	Rose is	I'm dreaming of
wait for	a rose is	of a
for	is	White Christmas
no man	a rose	

Now review your crititcal statements. Did you write about the errors in each phrase? Or did you ignore the errors and focus intstead on the content where your expectations suggested you look? Prehaps you also did not see the errors in this paragraph because you expected to see none.

THE ART OF READING

Reading is the main avenue by which you gather verbal information, so it goes without saying that you should be a good reader. This means being able to read a lot quickly and understand what you are reading. The act of reading involves moving the eye along the lines of text, translating the letters seen into sounds and words (phonics), and understanding the words being read. Most of us are adequate at the phonics stage but not as good as we could be in terms of our eye movements and comprehension.

The eye takes in most clearly material that is directly in front of it. As the eye moves along the written line, different parts of the line are brought into focus, and the eye stops for just a second to absorb that image. At each stopping point, or fixation, the eye of the average reader takes in three or four words, making three to six fixations per line. While the brain processes this information, the eye, a jump ahead, moves on to the next fixation point. Sometimes, the eye will backtrack to look again at previously read material. In addition to the material straight ahead of it, the eye can also make out images to the sides in what is known as peripheral vision. The brain uses peripheral vision to anticipate what is coming next.

Speed reading courses increase your speed by training you to take in more words at each fixation point, cut down the number of fixations needed per line, eliminate the tendency to regress, and make more use of peripheral vision. An average reader can cover between 250 to 300 words per minute, although not necessarily with complete comprehension, while a good reader will maintain that rate with full comprehension. Speed reading courses aim to increase your speed to 2,000 words per minute or more. While most of us can profitably learn to read faster and with better comprehension, the very rapid speeds are more suitable for skimming material than for reading with complete understanding. To read to best advantage, it is good to be able to read quickly, but you should modify your rate according to the purpose for which you are reading and the difficulty of the text. You can learn skimming techniques at a speed reading course, or you can do it independently by following through on a speed reading program outlined in a number of books. You might try the program developed by Norman Maberly in *Mastering Speed Reading*, a Signet paperback.

Scanning is a technique akin to skimming and is useful in providing you with a quick overview of material. It comes in handy for checking out all those extra news items and magazine articles we mentioned before. To scan an article, read the headline and the subheadings. Then glance through the various paragraphs and, if you want to learn a bit more, pick up the key phrases. When you are scanning an article, it is good to keep in mind that most follow the same pattern. The first paragraph usually presents a summary of what the article is about and the succeeding paragraphs provide the details in ever-increasing intricacy as you go down the page. So, after getting the main idea, go further only if you are truly interested.

Most people get through novels easily, but obviously it is more difficult to understand technical, philosophical, and scientific texts, or material in a field about which we know little. Understanding what you read can be facilitated in a number of ways. First, get an overview of the material. As in scanning, you want to get a quick look at titles and subheadings. In reading a short article, there is not much difference between scanning and an overview, but if you are reading a book, there is more to take in. Check the table of contents so you have an idea of the material to be covered and the layout of the book. Some chapters may be more important and some may be less important to you. Next, flip through the pages for visual material such as photos, drawings, diagrams. Highlights and summaries of the material are often presented graphically, because that format is easier to absorb. The blurb on the book cover or jacket will also give you a perspective on the book and perhaps even a summary of the material contained in it. Step two in reading a book is to turn through the pages rapidly and read all section and subsection headings, eye-catching material—such as boldfaced print or sections in italics—and all the summary sections. When you are finished with step two, ask yourself what you have read. Can you repeat to yourself the topics covered in the chapters and the main ideas presented? If not, go back and review the sections of the book you had difficulty with once more. When you can comfortably recall the main points of the chapters, you can do one of two things. If the book is not that interesting to you and you have no need to read it, you can put it aside and be done with it. If you are interested or are required to read it through, you are ready to begin. This may sound like a complicated and time-consuming way to read a book, but it is actually more efficient. Because you have a good idea at the outset about what you are going to read and a framework on which to hang the ideas the book contains, you will be able to read with more understanding and reduce the time you would ordinarily spend in going back over material that you couldn't grasp. Also, because you have an overview of the book and a mental outline of the contents, you will be able to save time by skipping over sections that you have already discovered are unimportant, repetitive, or previously familiar to you.

When it comes to books, people tend either to treat them as work tools that can be written in and marked up, or as treasures that should not be marred in any way. If you are of the latter type, it may be difficult to change your attitude, but you will probably get more out of your books if you are ready to mark them up. Underlining and bracketing improve your comprehension of material that is difficult to understand. The purpose of underlining is not to make phrases stand out when you reread or review a book, but to improve your comprehension while you are reading. The process of underscoring, especially in different colors for different concepts, helps to underscore the idea in your mind at the same time.

If you are not reading a murder mystery that you cannot put down until the end, it is a good idea to take a reading break every half-hour or so—longer or shorter depending on how well the break corresponds to a chapter ending or some other sensible division. The break allows you time to rest your eyes and to review the material in your mind. Go over what you have read and repeat the highlights to yourself. This improves your understanding and it also will do wonders for your ability to remember the material.

NOTES AND MIND MAPS

Note-taking is a prime occupation of students trying to master difficult verbal material. Actually, most people take notes, whether of a lecture, a business meeting, or a book, as an aid in remembering the material, but note-taking is important in understanding the material as well. Not all books are well written or well organized and taking notes can be a way of reordering the material so it becomes more sensible. As you organize the material for your notebook, you are also getting to understand it better. The value of note-taking lies in increasing your comprehension. When you take notes, keep the following points in mind: Notes should be brief, clear, and crisp. Write your notes in outline form, underline main topics, indent for subsidiary ideas, and put the main thoughts first. Limit your notes to key words and phrases. If you want a transcript of a lecture, take a tape recorder with you, but use your notes for jotting down central themes and critical ideas. Similarly, when you take notes from a book, you don't want to reproduce long paragraphs from it. Take notes that organize and highlight the main points of the book. To give you an example, if we wanted to take notes on the previous section on reading, we could do it this way:

> READING:
> Increase Speed
>   Perceptual span
>
> Scanning
>   Headings, subheadings
>   First paragraph
>
> Comprehension
>   Overview

Comprehension, *continued*

        Section headings, summaries, eye-catchers
        Playback chapters
        Underline
        Rest and review

Another method akin to note-taking is making mind maps, a process described in more detail by Tony Buzan in his book *Use Both Sides of Your Brain*. Map-making means, essentially, making visual rather than verbal notes. The value of mind maps is that they have higher memory value than words alone, since people are generally better at recalling visual images than verbal material (see the chapter, "Improving Memory"). Obviously then, the more visual the map, the more memory value it has. Maps done in color and with drawings are more effective than those using words, but we won't give you such a dramatic example here, being restricted to black ink and standard typefaces. Nevertheless, here is a mind map covering the same material on reading as was presented in note form above.

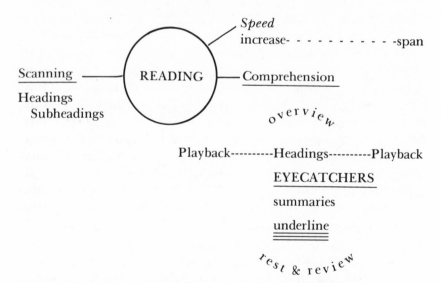

If you want to make a map, here are some pointers:

1. Draw the material in a map that reflects how the ideas and thoughts are related to each other
2. Use key words and short phrases
3. Better yet, whenever possible, represent the key ideas in a

visual image or print the words in distinctive ways that reflect
the same concept:

BIG   little   T
                                                             A
                                                             L
                                                             L

4. Connect your pictures/words with lines that show how they
   are connected conceptually. Use arrows where appropriate,
   bold lines for strong connections, weak lines for weak connections, etc.

5. Use lots of color, both to make the ideas stand out and to help
   you remember them later.

You'll find that map-making is fun and gets you so involved that
you'll have trouble getting your maps out of your mind.

ALGORITHMS

Very often verbal material seems hard to understand because it is
presented in an unclear or complicated fashion. Complicated
wording can become overwhelming when there is a series of
steps to follow and they are all unclear. Although the bureau-
crats responsible for government forms, insurance contracts,
credit card agreements and the like are becoming aware of the
difficulty people face in understanding their documents, little
progress has been made in simplifying them. This is where
algorithms come in.

"Algorithm" simply means an orderly sequence of instructions. Algorithms reduce complex tasks to a series of simple
steps, each one usually involving the choice between two alternatives. These alternatives can be set out diagrammatically to
simplify the task even further. The following examples are all
taken from actual documents, with the names deleted to protect
the guilty. The following paragraph comes from a TV warranty:

> The warranty herein extends only to the original consumer pur-
> chaser and is not assignable or transferable and shall not apply to
> any receiver or parts or transistors or tubes thereof which have

been repaired or replaced by anyone else other than an authorized dealer, service contractor or distributor, or which have been subject to alteration, misuse, negligence or accident, or to the parts or tubes or transistors of any receiver which have had the serial number or name altered, defaced or removed.

To simplify the warranty conditions, we'll lay them out a step at a time, putting each in the form of a question, with the alternatives for each question clearly diagrammed:

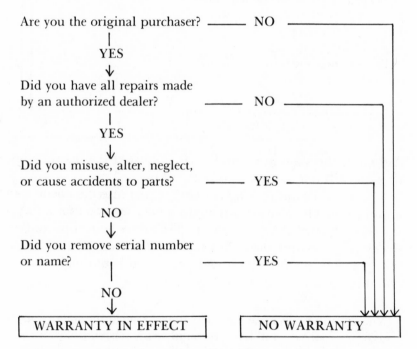

If you chart the steps as you read through instructions, you will find the time saved in trying to understand the text is usually a great deal more than the time required to write out the algorithm, and the results will be clearer, by eliminating confusion.

Here is another example of poorly written instructions taken from an old state income tax return form.

You must file a return if you are required to file a federal return and even though you may not be required to file a federal return you must nevertheless file this return if you meet any one of the following three conditions.

Putting this into simplified form, we end up with this algorithm:

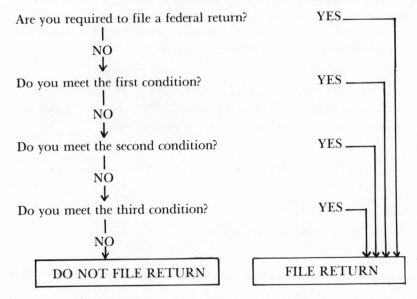

Although the state in question has improved the instructions, they are still not as clear as our algorithm.

This third example is taken from a guaranteed student loan application. The instructions are so poorly written that we were not sure whether it was intended to discourage loan applicants or to act as a screening device for college: if you could not make it out, you did not belong in college; if you could make it out, you did not need to go to college.

> You have to begin repaying your student loan at the end of your grace period. You will have to complete the repayment arrangements with your lender before the end of your grace period so you will know the amount of your payment and the length of your repayment period. Those arrangements will be written into your installment note. The minimum acceptable payment is $50 per month. You do not have to begin repaying your loan until your grace period is ended, and you will have not less than 5 years to repay the loan in full. But if the amount you owe would result in a monthly payment that is less than $50 a month you will have to pay at least $50 a month and repay the loan in less than 5 years. Your repayment period can not be more than 10 years. You will repay in monthly installments beginning at the end of your grace period. Your payments must be at least $50 per month or $600 per year, but they can be more depending on how much you borrowed. If the

loan is disbursed on or after October 1, 1981, notwithstanding the other provisions of this loan, the lender may require a repayment period shorter than 5 years if this is necessary to ensure that during each year of the repayment period you pay toward the principal and interest at least $600 or the unpaid balance, whichever is less, of the total amount owing.

Laying out this paragraph in algorithmic form yields the following instructions:

		Minimum Payment	*Minimum Years*
Does amount owed involve payments of less than $50 month/ $600 year?	YES ⟶	$50 month/$600 year	less than 5
	NO ⟶	$50 month/$600 year	5 years
Was your loan disbursed after October 31, 1981?	YES ⟶	$50 month/$600 year	number required at that rate
	NO ⟶	$50 month/$600 year	5 years

It quickly becomes obvious on looking at the algorithm that the paragraph could have simply stated that everyone has to pay the loan back with minimum monthly payments of fifty dollars and that at this rate some persons will repay their loan before five years are up while others will have a repayment period of more than five years because they borrowed more.

The next time you are faced with poorly written material that is needlessly complicated, try putting it in algorithmic form. You might even offer your algorithm to the firm, bureau, or individual responsible for the confusing text so that it could be used to benefit others.

ORDERING INFORMATION

The way information is presented to us influences how well we can understand and use it. Certain orders of presentation appear to us more natural than others. We are geared to specific progressions: from first to last, from big to small, from good to bad, from above to below, and so on. When information is presented to us out of these sequences as, for example, from last to first or from small to big, we usually find it much more difficult to take in.

From your daily life experiences you know that your first impressions are stronger than your subsequent impressions. How often have you been disappointed in people because, as you got to know them well they turned out to be so different from what you first thought them to be? Probably the reverse has happened to you as well: someone you did not like right away because your first impressions were unfavorable turned out to be nice after all. This same process works on all information that we come across: the material we see first has a greater impact than what follows.

Exercise

Cross out the one word on each line that does not belong with the other three.

skyscraper   cathedral   temple   prayer

thyme   garlic   chives   daffodils

factory   laboratory   dormitory   books

undershirt   blouse   vest   hat

Chances are your answers and reasoning were as follows:

skyscraper, cathedral, and *temple* are all buildings; cross out *prayer,* which does not belong.

thyme, garlic, and *chives* are all herbs; cross out *daffodils,* which are flowers.

factory, laboratory, and *dormitory* are all buildings in which people congregate; cross out *books,* which does not belong.

undershirt, blouse, and *vest* are all garments for the midbody; cross out *hat,* which goes on the head.

Exercise

Here are the same groups of words, but with their order changed. The task is the same. Cross out the one word that does not belong with the other three.

prayer   cathedral   temple   skyscraper

daffodils   garlic   chives   thyme

books   laboratory   dormitory   factory

hat   blouse   vest   undershirt

You will notice that the order of presentation can make a decisive difference in how you interpret the relationship between words:

prayer, cathedral and *temple* belong together because they are related to religious observance; now *skyscraper* does not fit in.

daffodils, garlic, and *chives* are all bulbs, and *thyme* is the plant that does not belong.

books, laboratory, and *dormitory* are all education and college-related, but *factory* does not fit in.

hat, blouse, and *vest* are all outer garments, and *undershirt* is the word that does not belong.

Just by repositioning the words you see first and last, your understanding of a whole group of words can change. Keep in mind the natural tendency to be influenced by the first thing you see and try not to let it get in your way of accurately processing information.

Now let's examine some of the other naturally favored orders of presentation. Look, for example, at the two sets of statements below:

1

A is better than B
B is better than C

2

C is worse than B
B is worse than A

Both sets of statements mean essentially the same thing, but set 1 is easier to understand than set 2. The reason is that we grasp information best when we can visualize it, and certain orders of presentation make information easier to visualize than others. Generally, we do best with information that we can imagine in a vertical line going from top to bottom or in a horizontal line going from left to right, these directions being the ones we use when we read. The statements "A is better than B" and "B is better than C" let us visualize A first, with B below it, and C underneath B. The statements "C is worse than B" and "B is worse than A" can only be visualized if we start with C and put B above it, and then put A above B, thus reversing the natural order. Just as it is easier to deal with information in the form of "better" rather than "worse," you will find it easier to deal with "bigger" rather than "smaller," "taller" rather than "shorter," "higher" rather than "lower," and so on, because these forms can be visualized in a line going down or in a line going from left to right. This means that when you are dealing with information presented to you in an unnatural sequence, the best way to process it is to change it to a natural order. Going back to set 2 above, we can change the statements.

from	*to*	*and then to*
C is worse than B	B is better than C	A is better than B
B is worse than A	A is better than B	B is better than C

In the everyday world we don't usually deal with ABCs, so let's see how the principle works in a more usual example. Suppose you were reading the following information:

"The population of Cincinnati, Ohio, is smaller than that of Cleveland, Ohio, and the population of Akron is smaller than that of Cincinnati."

You will absorb this information much better if you switch it around, as follows:

"The population of Cleveland, Ohio is larger than the population of Cincinnati, Ohio, and the population of Cincinnati, Ohio, is larger than that of Akron, Ohio. . . ."

Often, when collecting information, you will find that not only is it presented in an unnatural form and order, which you will want to change, but that the order is inconsistent. Consider the following example:

C is worse than B
A is better than B

The first step necessary to make this information easier to understand is to put it in consistent form:

C is worse than B = B is better than C
A is better than B = A is better than B

Then reorder it in a natural progression:

A is better than B
B is better than C

In reading, you might come across information of this type in the following way:

When we go metric, remember that a centimeter is less than an inch, a meter is more than a yard, and a kilometer is less than a mile.

It will be easier to grasp this information if you reorder it as follows:

When we go metric, remember that an inch is more than a centimeter, a meter is more than a yard, and a mile is more than a kilometer.

DEALING WITH NEGATIVES

Most people find it quite difficult to deal with information presented in negative form. Here, for example, are two equivalent statements. One is presented in a positive form: "This page is printed in black ink." One is presented in a negative form: "This page is not printed in red ink." The positive statement can be processed much more readily than can the negative statement, and many find the negative statement hard to comprehend. Since a lot of information is presented in negative form, it is important that you understand the blocks to dealing with negative information and how to circumvent them. First, let's see how much trouble you currently have absorbing information in negative form.

Exercise

Below are two lists of statements. Your task is to write down after each whether it is true or false. Get yourself a stopwatch or timer. First do List A and note the time it takes you; then do list B and note the time it takes you.

List A

	True	False
21 is an even number	( )	( )
18 is an even number	( )	( )
12 is an odd number	( )	( )
15 is an even number	( )	( )
29 is an odd number	( )	( )

List B

	True	False
29 is not an even number	( )	( )
6 is not an odd number	( )	( )
18 is not an even number	( )	( )
33 is not an odd number	( )	( )
42 is not an even number	( )	( )

You probably found that List B took you longer to do than List A, because the statements in List B are all negatively phrased. The bigger the difference between the time you spent on List A and List B, the greater problem you have dealing with information in negative form. One reason it is more difficult to deal with negatives is that our learning patterns are usually positive. That is, we learn what things are, rather than what they are not. When teaching a child to recognize domestic animals, we will point to a four-legged creature and say, "This is a dog," rather than "This is not a cat." A negative statement ("This is not a cat") only makes sense if we already have the positive concept ("This *is* a cat"). Negatives are a transformation of a more basic idea or thought, namely, the positive idea. Another reason negative statements are more difficult to process than positive statements is that they tend to be emotionally loaded for us. We associate negatives with admonitions: "Don't do that"; "I said, NO," and so on.

Because statements in negative form are based on a denial of a positive idea, they are associated with the exceptional case. That is, we tend to use a negative expression to indicate an unusual condition. The statement "Harold is not on time today" implies that Harold usually is on time; the statement "The train did not stop at Forty-second Street" implies that the train usually does stop there, and so on. Negative statements thus arouse certain assumptions on our part, but these assumptions may not be valid. It is important for you to be aware of this tendency when you deal with negative information, to make sure you do not misinterpret it. The following exercise should help you in this regard.

Exercise

Match up the statements on the right side with the figures that illustrate the statements.

	Figures	Fill in correct figure #	Statements
(1)	☐☐☐☐	_____	(a) The third square does not contain an x.
(2)	☒☒☒☐	_____	(b) The left-end square does not contain an x.
(3)	☒☒☐☒	_____	(c) The right-end square does not contain an x.
(4)	☐☒☒☒	_____	(d) The two center squares do not contain an x.
(5)	☒☐☐☒	_____	(e) None of the squares contains a y.

For many people, the most obvious answers are those indicated in column 1, below. The answers in column 3, however, are also correct and just as valid as the answers in column 1.

Usual Answers	Statements	Other Correct Answers
Figure 3	The third square does not contain an x	Figures 1 and 5
Figure 4	The left-end square does not contain an x	Figure 1
Figure 2	The right-end square does not contain an x	Figure 1
Figure 5	The two center squares do not contain an x	Figures 1 and 3
Figure 1	None of the squares contains a y	Figures 2, 3, 4 and 5

Because negative statements are associated with the exceptional case rather than with the rule, we tend to overlook ordinary situations to which they apply. In statement (a) "the third square does not contain an x," we tend to interpret this as meaning "the third square is the *only* square that does not contain an x." We thus ignore Figures 1 and 5, where the third squares are also empty and do not contain an x. This same reasoning process makes us overlook other correct answers given in column 3.

Negatives also give us difficulty when we have too many of them. You cannot not make a mistake when you do not have many positive elements in a thought. To translate that last statement into simple English, the best procedure is to turn the negatives into positives:

You cannot |not make a mistake| = You cannot |be correct| when you|do not have many positive elements| = when you|have many negative elements|

Putting the translated phrases together, the sentence now reads: "You cannot be correct when you have many negative elements in a thought." When you have to deal with statements that are hard to understand because they contain multiple negatives, turn the negative phrases into positive phrases. Remember also that double negatives automatically become positive. Let's see how that works in the sentence we just used. The first part of that sentence has a double negative: "You *cannot not* make a mistake." We can bracket the double negative and replace it with a positive, as follows:

You |cannot not| make a mistake = You |can|make a mistake

Putting this phrase into the sentence preserves the same meaning as our previous translation: "You can make a mistake when you have many negative elements in a thought."

Exercise

Below are some statements in negative form. Try to make them more intelligible by converting the negative phrases into positive phrases or by turning the double negatives into positives.

If it was not the case that she was not going to the movies, he did not want to say no.

He is neither not tall nor not thin but he is not bad-looking.

If you are not unconscious you cannot be unaware of what is happening.

It is not true that she does not believe in God, but she is not irreligious.

If she doesn't not eat and doesn't stay not drunk she won't get depressed.

Here is another one from a stock-market advisory letter that recently came to our attention. See if you can figure it out. "At this point, none of the market averages have failed to hit a new rally high, so no non-confirmations have occurred."

ENHANCING PERCEPTION

Information about the world comes to us through our senses and serves as a foundation of our intelligence. If our perceptual systems do not function effectively, we are obviously hampered. Enhancing perceptual capabilities is, therefore, an important part of increasing intelligence.

Although we experience perception as an automatic process and take for granted that what we hear, touch, taste, and smell accurately informs us about the nature of the world, this is far from the way perception works. Our perceptions are not simple, direct reflections of what is out there, but interpretations made by our brain that are subject to various limitations and distortions. Even when our sensory organs are functioning properly, they register only a small spectrum of the actual data available. Our eyes respond only to a narrow band of light waves, our ears are deaf to very high and very low tones, and our other sensory systems are similarly limited. Further, the sensory data that we receive can be misinterpreted by the brain either because of the nature of the stimulus itself or because of our preconceptions and attitudes. We become so habituated to perceiving things in certain ways that we often fail to register information that does not fit in with our established framework. In this chapter we will look at the impediments to clear perception and how to overcome them.

SEEING AND BELIEVING

Sight is our most highly developed sense and the one on which we depend the most. Visual material accounts for roughly 90 percent of the brain's input of sensory material. The importance of sight in understanding what is going on around us is reflected in the language we use to describe intellectual experiences. We say, "I see" when we grasp an idea, and that "he has insight" when he can figure something out. People "have vision" when they can imaginatively project trends, and the word *imagination* is rooted in "image"—again a visual phenomenon. Despite our heavy reliance on sight, we do not make the best use of this sense, because several factors get in the way. What we see, or rather, what we think we see, is different from the image that falls on our eye.

What happens when we see something is that light waves, reflected by the various objects in front of us, enter the eye through the lens. The light is focused by the lens on the back of the eyeball, or retina, where it forms a representation in miniature of the outside scene that is reflecting the light. This retinal image, however, is not an exact copy. In addition to being greatly reduced in size from the original, it is two-dimensional rather than three-dimensional and, more surprisingly, the image is upside-down. If what hits our eye, then, is a small, flat, upside-down universe, how do we see the world the way it is? The best theory to date is that seeing takes place not in the eyes, but in the brain. As the brain receives visual information from the retinal cells, it utilizes other information already stored to make sense out of the distorted image being transmitted. We do not perceive what hits our eye, but learn to override what we see to get a better picture of what the world is really like. Whenever we see, there is a complex inter-action going on between retinal impulses and other nerve impulses produced by the brain. These interactions occur very quickly, because we have learned to develop habits of seeing and interpreting visual input. These habits are so set that we are not even aware of them.

One of the most important habits of perception is known as size constancy. When you look at a woman five feet tall who is standing in front of you, her image covers most of the retina, but as she walks twenty feet away her image covers much less of the retina. You do not, however, see the incredible shrinking woman, but a woman whose size is constant. Your brain has stored the information that a woman's size does not change when she moves, and so you can ignore the size of her image on your retina and use your experience to interpret what you see. The following experiments demonstrate how strong the size constancy habit is.

Experiment

For this experiment you need a full-sized pencil and a room ten to twelve feet in length. Enter the room and walk three feet in. Turn around and look back at the doorway. Now walk to the farthest end of the room and look at the doorway again. It probably looks the same size as it did before, about seven feet in height. Standing in the same spot, hold the pencil about twelve inches in front of one eye, close the other eye, and look at the pencil. Now, compare the length of the pencil with the height of the doorway. The seven-inch pencil looks bigger than the seven-foot doorway. This is because the pencil's image on your retina is bigger. Yet, when you looked at the doorway as you ordinarily do, without the pencil for comparison, it did not look smaller than a pencil, but seven feet high.

Experiment

This experiment utilizes the retina's tendency to create *afterimages*, caused by continual firing of the retina after stimulation. Do this experiment in a room ten to twelve feet long that is painted white or light-toned and has some uncluttered wall space. You will need an 8½ × 11 inch piece of white paper, and a black disc—a button, checker, licorice candy or cutout paper will do. Stand two feet away from one wall and ten to twelve feet away from another. Place the paper with black disc centered on it atop a table, chair, or other surface. Stare intently at the black disc and count to sixty. Then look up at the wall close by. You will see the afterimage of the disc as a round spot on the wall. (You might also see an afterimage of the paper surrounding it.) Now quickly look at the wall ten feet away from you. You will again see the round spot on the wall, but this time it will seem much larger. The reason for this apparent change in size is as follows: The impression on the retina remains the same size, but your distance from the wall that you have fixated upon changes. Experience has taught you that if two objects occupy the same area on the retina and one is farther away, then the more distant one must be larger. Thus you see the distant afterimage as larger.

When we see things at great distances, size constancy breaks down. For example, looking out of an airplane window at the ground below, the cars seem as small as toys and the buildings like miniature models. Size constancy also breaks down when we are not familiar with the objects involved. In order to interpret size correctly despite changes in retinal size, we have to have had experience with the object.

In addition to size constancy, we also have the habits of shape, brightness, and position constancy. Just as the retinal image of objects changes as they are viewed at different distances, their retinal shape changes when viewed at different angles, their retinal brightness changes when viewed in different illuminations, and their retinal image shifts as we move our eyes or bodies. Yet, we manage to see things as constant in shape, brightness, and position. To illustrate shape constancy, take a penny from your pocket. If you look at the penny head on, a circular shape appears on your retina and if you look at it from its side, an elliptical shape appears on your retina. Regardless of which way you view it, however, you still see a circle.

One of the difficulties many children have when beginning to read is based on shape constancy. They frequently confuse b, d, and p because they see these three letters as one basic shape. The change in orientation does not signal to them a different object any more than a penny turned on its side looks like a different object. As with size constancy, shape constancy depends on familiarity with the object involved. If you were to rotate an unfamiliar form in space, its shape constancy would be disrupted because a constancy "habit" would not have been established.

The brightness constancy habit allows you to recognize the identity of objects when they are viewed under different light. When you look at this page in daylight, for example, the retinal image is white, but if you were to read it in twilight the retinal image would be gray. We nevertheless see a white page under both conditions.

The habit of position constancy develops because you have learned to discount the moving images that impinge on your eyes when you move and the world stands still. Suppose that you move your eyes across the room. Even though the retina now receives moving images of furniture and bric-a-brac, you see the room as stable. A different habit comes into play when you see movement. If you follow a moving object with your eyes, the image on your retina remains more or less stationary. You still see movement, however, even though the retinal image cannot signal movement. Your brain interprets movement of the object from the movement of your eyes. We are not aware of the fact that we are interpreting what we see and setting images right. Our brains make allowances for what we see, enabling us to respond to the constant properties of objects. Our perceptions are not the patterns that fall on the retina, but interpretations produced by the brain, based on our experience with the size, shape, and spatial relationships of objects.

Underlying our interpretation of retinal images to reflect a world of constant physical objects is the ability to perceive those objects in the first place. When reflecting light waves hit our eyes they do not come labeled as to what they represent or where their boundaries are. Yet we see the tree as distinct from the ground and the perched bird as distinct from the tree. Moreover, we do not see a trunk, branches, and leaves as discrete objects, but we see a tree, just as we do not see feathers, beak, and claws, but a bird. We interpret light waves as representing distinct but meaningful objects.

The tendency of the brain to create coherent visual images from the retinal stimuli it receives sometimes leads us to see things that are not reflected on the eye at all, as well as at other times *not* to see things that are visible. At the point on the retina, for example, where blood vessels enter and fibers exit to form the optic nerve, we all have a blind spot. This means that whatever we look at we see with a hole in it, but the brain fills in this blind spot so that we interpret objects to be whole rather than holed. You can check out your own blind spot with a simple experiment.

Experiment

Hold a pencil at arm's length against a backdrop of a blank wall. Close one eye and fixate at a spot just above the pencil tip. Keeping your eye on that same spot, slowly move the pencil away from you and out of your line of vision. You will notice that the pencil tip suddenly disappears and then reappears again as it reaches the outer limit of your visual field. When the tip of the pencil disappears it is because the light waves reflecting from the tip are falling on your blind spot. Ordinarily you are not aware of this visual hole, but fill in the missing spots.

In addition to seeing what is not there, your mind also tends not to see what is there that gets in the way. The retina, for example, is fed by small blood vessels which, being on the surface of the eye, are visible. We don't usually see them because the brain chooses to ignore them as not part of the scene in front of us. What we consciously perceive, therefore, fits in with our interpretation of what the world is like. The problem is, we don't always make the correct interpretation. Because our perceptual habits are so well developed, we can not easily shake them and we automatically bring them to bear, even when not called for. We are thus prone to a variety of perceptual traps. Knowing how you can get tripped up will help you to be more alert and to avoid these pitfalls.

PERCEPTUAL TRAPS

Size Constancy and Distance

When we develop our constancy habits we learn, unconsciously, about a series of relationships between retinal images and the objects they represent. We learn, as the experiments showed, the relationship between retinal size and distance and also how to estimate distance. By experience we come to know that objects in the distance seem smaller, less distinct in contour, and less bright. We also learn that near objects seem to obscure more distant ones and that lines seem to converge as they move into the distance. Painters have developed these relationships into the art of perspective. They can create the illusion of depth and distance by texture gradients, shadows, brightness differences, obscuring of one object by another, varying size differences, and converging lines. When we look at a traditional landscape painting we get the illusion of depth, but we still know it is a two-dimensional canvas. Many times, however, what we have learned about perspective and the relationship between retinal images and objects serves to deceive us. This is what can happen in the case of visual illusions. Ordinarily we have to override our retinal images to make correct interpretations, but in the case of illusions, bypassing the retinal image leads to incorrect interpretations.

One of the most famous illusions is that developed by Müller-Lyer:

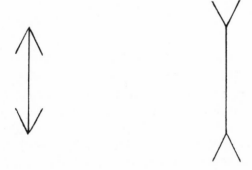

Although both lines are equal, people invariably perceive the one on the right as longer—in this country, that is. Susceptibility to the Müller-Lyer illusion varies by culture. It is strongest in societies where people live in an environment of right-angled edges (such as building corners) and are used to perspective cues to distance such as the converging lines of roads and railways. In cultures where right-angled objects don't exist, and even the houses are round, such as the Zulu of Africa, or in cultures where distance cannot be visually experienced, as in dense forest cultures, the illusion does not hold. Imagine that the two drawings below, a slight modification of the Müller-Lyer illusion, represent parts of buildings. The one on the left looks like the outside corner of a building, and the one on the right like the inside corner of a room.

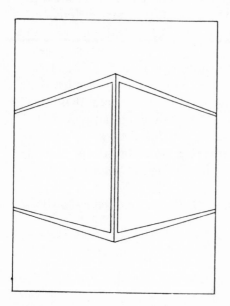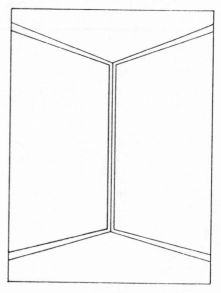

The outside corner seems to be approaching us while the inner corner seems to be receding. Experience tells us that the retinal size of a receding object shrinks and that of an approaching one grows. Thus, although the two corner lengths are equal, the size constancy habit causes us to perceive the receding corner as larger. If it is further away and equal in size on the retina, we conclude it must be larger. Had we not built up this perceptual habit because of our visual environment, we would not make the mistake that we do.

Other incorrect interpretations can be created by utilizing our perceptual habits regarding perspective.

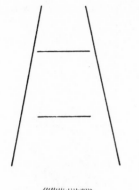

Here the upper horizontal line looks larger than the lower line because it is enclosed in a narrower space.

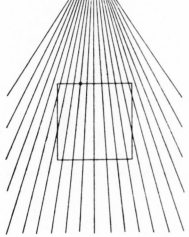

Here the square appears to be a distorted figure, wider at the top, because of our tendency to see the whole image receding into the distance.

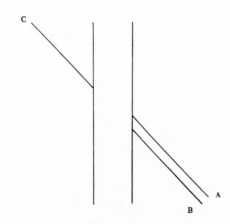

The diagonal line appears to run from A to C, whereas it runs from B to C. This shift occurs, apparently, because the upper segment of the line appears to be receding into the distance, causing it to shift visually upward.

Surroundings

Because we make perceptual judgments of objects in relation to their surroundings, we can also be misled into incorrect perceptual interpretations when those surroundings are manipulated. Look at the following illustrations:

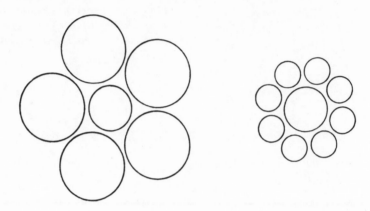

The circle surrounded by smaller circles looks larger than the circle surrounded by larger circles, although both are equal in size.

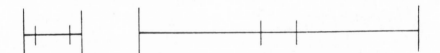

The line segment in the middle looks bigger when it is enclosed in a smaller space.

The tendency to be led astray by cues in the surroundings also functions to create misperceptions of brightness, as in the following experiment.

Experiment

Cut out one-inch squares of black, light gray, and white construction paper, and three ½-inch squares of dark gray paper. Paste the ½-inch dark gray squares in the center of each of the larger squares. Arrange the three large squares on a table about six inches apart. Now have a friend look at the squares and tell you which of the small squares is the darkest and which is the lightest. You will find that the small squares, although all the same, seem to get increasingly darker to the observer as the background gets increasingly lighter.

Directionals

Directional signals can create illusions because of the tendency of the eye to follow a line. The illustration below makes this point very clearly.

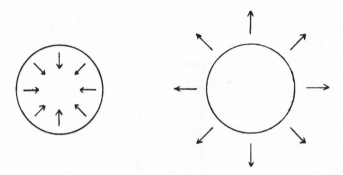

The circle on the right looks considerably larger than the one on the left because we follow the arrows with our eyes, creating the impression of an enlarged circle.

The effect of following directional signals works just as effectively in enclosed areas. Look at the two squares below:

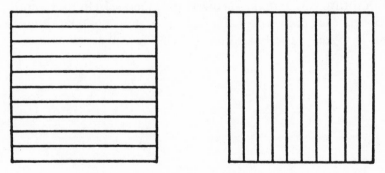

Neither of these two equal squares appears to be a square. The left one is seen to be wider than it is high, an illusion created by the horizontal filler, while the right one is seen to be taller than it is wide, an illusion created by the vertical filler.

The second illustration shows why fashion experts counsel heavy people to wear vertically striped garments and to avoid horizontals. As the eye is led to follow the up-down dimension it is diverted from noticing the width and breadth of a person. Interior decorators also follow this principle when they create the illusion of a higher ceiling in a room by using vertically striped wallpaper, or when they reduce the impression of height by using a horizontal pattern.

Position

Which looks longer in the picture below—the height of the hat or its brim?

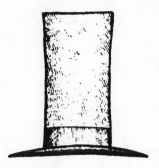

As you probably have guessed by now, the dimensions are equal, even though the hat looks taller than it is wide. If you look at the following series of line pairs, you can see the effect of position on prompting you to make incorrect judgments. In figures 1 and 2, it appears that the vertical line is longer than the horizontal line, but in figure 3 the horizontal line looks longer:

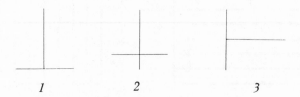

Thus, the illusion of greater length does not depend on whether the line is vertical as opposed to horizontal. The reason our judgments get distorted appears to be the fact that one line seems to interrupt another. In the three illustrations above, the line that sits atop or cuts through the other line appears to be longer. If two lines equally intersect each other, so that neither is an interrupter, the illusion disappears (Figures 4 & 5).

4   *5*

Empty Space

Distance and area are misperceived depending on whether they are empty or filled spaces. When space is filled it appears greater than when it is empty. To test this out, try the following experiment.

Experiment

Draw three dots in a line, one inch apart. Fill in the right-hand space with a series of dots. Now look at the two spaces. The one that is filled looks larger than the equal but empty space.

Although empty space appears smaller than filled space, half-enclosures appear bigger than complete enclosures, as the following illustration shows:

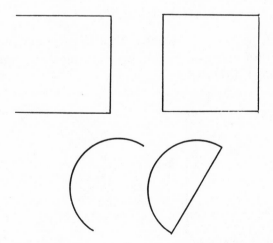

The openness invites us to enlarge upon the contours, while the closed figures clearly define the boundaries.

Brightness

Bright light creates a spreading effect, making us perceive light objects as larger than dark ones. Look at the two figures below.

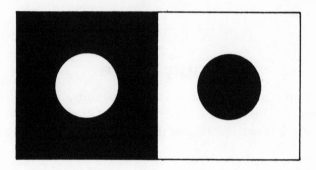

The white circle probably appears larger than the black one. This illusion is also important in fashion. People who want to create a smaller impression are well-advised to wear dark clothes. "Basic black" has a good deal to recommend it. Although you may want to package yourself to look thin, manufacturers who want you to think you are getting more for your money stick to bright colors to create the illusion of greater size.

Imbedding

Sometimes, apparent distortions in figures can be created by the shapes and lines within them or surrounding them. Some illustrations of this follow below.

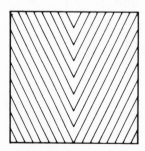

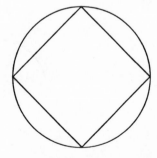

This square appears to become wider at the bottom.

This is a perfect circle that appears flattened by the square inside.

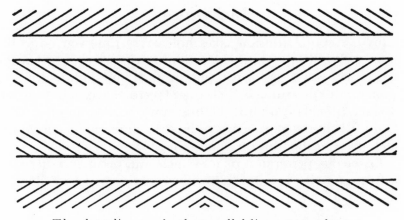

The short lines make the parallel lines appear bent.

Superimposition of shape and lines can also cause distortion.

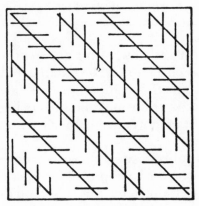

The long lines are parallel to each other but do not appear so because of the short lines crossing them.

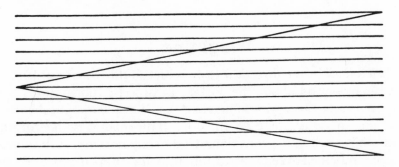

The sides of the angle, although made of straight lines, appear twisted by the parallel lines.

Movement

This perceptual illusion takes hold every time you go to the movies. While you enjoy the action on the screen, all that the retina sees is a series of still photos, each one slightly different from the one preceding it, flicked at 24 pictures a second (or, for an average film, 115,200 still pictures run one after another). The brain fills in the gaps between the stills to maintain continuity and give you the illusion of movement.

Erroneous perception of movement can occur in other situations as well. Try the following experiment to see illusory movement.

Experiment

Place a small flashlight or a lighted cigarette in an ashtray at the far end of a completely dark room. Have a friend enter the room and stare at the light for a count of ten. The light will seem to move, swaying back and forth and/or swooping in one direction.

The best theory as to why this apparent movement occurs is that the eyes become fatigued by fixating and require command signals to continue the fixation; because these same signals also cause the eye to fixate on and follow a moving object, the signals induce the effect of movement even when applied to prevent eye movement.

Movement is also misinterpreted because of the relationship between objects. You have probably experienced this yourself when seated on a train. Sometimes it is hard to know if your train is moving forward or if the one you see out the window is moving backward. Generally, when we see movement, we assume that it is the small object that is moving.

Lighting

Differences in the direction from which light comes can lead to misperceptions about the surface of objects. Indentations can appear to be protrusions and vice versa. The position of shadows on the surface creates these illusions. If the shadow is underneath, the object is seen to protrude and if the shadow is above, the object looks indented. We seem to fall into this trap because of our experience with light sources. We are used to light—sunlight and indoor light—coming from above. Under these conditions, a protrusion on a flat surface will be shadowy on the bottom and illuminated at the top.

Figure-Ground Relationship

We have seen that the sensory information that we receive is not accepted on its own, but is interpreted in relation to other information we have available to us. We develop the best perception, or hypothesis, to fit the data. Sometimes, it happens that equally good interpretations compete with each other, as in the case of certain ambiguous figures where we cannot really decide what we are seeing. As we look at such figures, we tend to switch back and forth between two possibilities, as in the following illustrations.

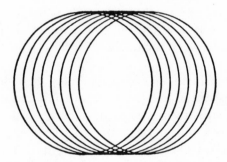

The rings appear to be a hollow tube running alternately from left to right or from right to left.

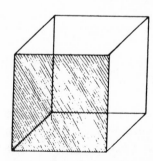

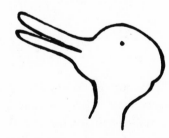

The shaded surface appears alternately like the outer surface of the box, facing front, or the interior.

This looks alternately like a duck facing left or a rabbit facing right.

In the three illustrations above we tend to stay open—switching back and forth between two equally good perceptions. Often, however, we tend to get trapped into viewing ambiguous figures as fixed. This happens when part of the illustration appears to be the figure and the other part the background on which it rests. Take the following illustration for example. Most people see black shapes on the white page. Try now to focus on the white and see the letters formed in the white space between the black:

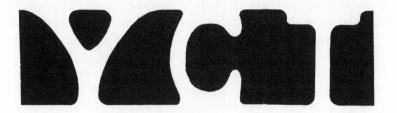

If you have trouble seeing the letters, just pencil in two horizontal lines across the tops and bottoms of the black shapes, including the white space between them. Now the letters Y C T will emerge clearly.

Several factors influence your tendency to be able to see one part of an illustration as figure rather than ground. As we saw with the Y C T illustration, an important determinant is contour. Figures that are contour-rich, and therefore spatially isolated, have a better chance of being seen as the figure. Smaller objects are similarly favored over big ones, brighter ones over duller ones, warmer-colored ones (red, orange) over cooler-colored ones (blue and green), moving over stationary ones, and odd ones over more usual ones.

IMPROVING PERCEPTION

Visual perception, or what you think you see, is a combination of what your eye takes in and how your brain interprets those sensations. So far we have looked at how our perceptual habits can draw us into making incorrect interpretations. But there are ways to improve perceptual technique to facilitate making correct interpretations. Whenever we look at something, we are making a decision, conscious or otherwise, as to where to look, what to focus on, and what it means. By becoming more deliberate in these functions, we can go a long way in improving the accuracy of our perceptions.

Looking

Whenever you open your eyes and look, you automatically focus on the most novel objects in front of you. From babyhood on our attention is drawn to the complex rather than the simple. Because of this tendency to focus on the unusual, you have to train yourself to take in a broader view. It will require conscious effort at first to make deliberate searches of your visual field, but after a while it will become habitual. Visually scanning your environment will not only provide you with a fuller picture of what is going on, but help your mind to stay alert.

Some things we do require us to shift our focus continually to many different targets. When you drive a car, for example, you have to watch the road in front, the rear-view mirror for traffic behind, the speedometer to see you are not speeding, the road signs to catch your highway exit, and perhaps the child sitting on the seat next to you. You cannot look at all these things at once, but you will be able to monitor them all to best advantage if you plan for them. Experienced drivers have this strategy so well worked out that it is automatic. When you are in new situations it can be helpful to map out beforehand what you have to look at and perhaps even roughly how long you should look before shifting your focus.

Another reason for frequently shifting your focus is to avoid fixation. If you look too long at any one thing you stop really seeing it. Prolonged fixation leads to inattention. If you are in a car this can cause accidents; in other situations, although physical danger may not be involved, it means you might miss out on something happening around you.

People also have a tendency to look at whatever they are thinking about. If, for example, you are at a party and the person you are talking to mentions someone else's name, say Mr. X., your eyes will automatically go to Mr. X. If your friend keeps talking about Mr. X., even though Mr. X. has moved away, you will probably keep fixating on the space where he was standing before. Looking at blank space does not provide you with any useful information, so be aware of this habit in order to break it and let your eyes wander.

When people are thinking about something that is present they will fixate on it, but what happens when they are thinking about something that is not present? In this case, they do not look straight ahead but characteristically look either to the right or the left. People usually follow handedness in this regard: right-handed people look to the right and left-handed people look to the left. There is also a tendency for all people to look to the left when solving a spatial problem and to look to the right when solving a verbal problem. Again, the looking in either direction does not add anything since you are not focusing on any particularly useful visual information. It can, though, interfere with your picking up visual cues if you keep your eyes fastened in one direction.

Analyzing

The first step in perception is sensory registration: an image falls on your retina. After that your perceptual habits go to work automatically to make sense of what your eyes take in. If you are not alert during this phase, you can fall into various sorts of perceptual traps. Giving your conscious attention to visual material will not only increase the probability of making a correct interpretation, but it will also facilitate your being able to store this information in your memory for future use.

To make the best use of what you perceive, it is helpful to label it, categorize it, and relate it to other information already accumulated. In most everyday situations, such analysis is relatively simple. When you walk down the street, for example, you ordinarily label your sensory images as people, cars, shops, traffic lights, and so forth. You might, depending on your interests and needs at the moment, make this categorizing more specific. That is, you might label the people as women and men, the cars by their manufacturers, the stores by their products or function, and so on. In many situations, however, organizing what we see into meaningful categories is harder to do because we are faced with unfamiliar material for which we do not yet have labels. Making meaningful perceptual judgments in these situations will be easier if you follow some organizing principles.

Grouping

To begin, try to group the unfamiliar visual material into simpler units. You already have a built-in tendency to do so, but you will perceive more efficiently if you maximize this tendency. Look at the following illustration.

. . . .

. . . .

. . . .

. . . .

. . . .

. . . .

Obviously, you see dots. But you probably immediately organized these dots into groups: either rows or columns of dots. The dots make more sense to you when they fall into a pattern. If the pattern is not immediately there, as in the example above, your job is to search out some organizing pattern by which the material can be made more coherent. In this instance, the pattern was obtained by finding simpler units. One of the best examples of this is the heavenly constellations, a legacy from ancient civilizations. Our ancestors looked at the skies and, in an effort to bring order to the multitude of otherwise random stars, patterned them into constellations. Knowing what the constellations are enables us to discern the groups, but first someone had to do that grouping. Of course, the grouping principles were sensible and fit the material, or they would not have endured for so long.

Two essential principles of grouping are proximity and similarity. If objects are too far apart or too dissimilar they lose their cohesion. The Big Dipper makes sense because the individual stars are close enough to belong together visually, and they are all more or less similar enough in size and brightness to impress us as elements of one common unit. They form a distinct pattern because they are spatially isolated from other stars, standing out as a figure upon the ground of the sky. In addition, none of the stars in the Big Dipper is pulled away by other nearby stars with which it could also be grouped. Still one more factor makes it possible for the Big Dipper to endure as a meaningful image— and that is already implied by its name. Meaningful perceptual units can be created out of otherwise meaningless material if they can be labeled as something familiar and similar in form.

Labeling

In naming unfamiliar visual material, the label, if it is to be of any use, has to help us understand the material better and therefore it has to fit the material. The Big Dipper is an example of good labeling because the constellation actually looks like a dipper. The constellation Orion has a less suitable label: looking at it one does not clearly see a man, although once the components are pointed out it is possible for the eye to fill in the rest and thereby perceive a pattern rather than an unrelated scattering of stars.

Not too long ago, the process of perceptual labeling was turned into a popular parlor game called "Droodles." Various drawings of seemingly meaningless and unrelated lines were presented to the reader, who was then supposed to guess (label) what they represented. Here are two such drawings. If you try to describe them as groups of lines it would be difficult to do, and they would be hard to remember, but if you label them, they become easy to describe and stand out on the page with great clarity:

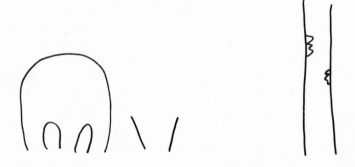

The drawing on the left is a kneeling woman scrubbing the floor, with her pail next to her (seen from behind). The drawing on the right is a bear climbing up a tree (seen from the other side). The process of labeling brings order into something that is otherwise quite meaningless to you, making it easier to remember and manipulate mentally.

One of the reasons many people do not like modern art is because the works frequently have no labels that communicate meaning. Nonrepresentational art is difficult for them to code in a way that the brain can store. For those people, such art is seen but not perceived, or really taken in.

Differentiating

When you are dealing with new visual material, it is helpful to look for its distinctive features. Differentiating among objects in the visual field requires a directed search and improves with experience. It is easy for us to look at the sky during the migratory period and label that moving cluster of black shapes as birds, but it requires more effort and experience to look at those clusters and see ducks or Canadian geese. Hunters, of course, learn to differentiate the distinctive characteristics of the various edible species, and bird fanciers learn to differentiate the distinctive characteristics of all species. Similarly you may look at the sky and see a plane, whereas a pilot would look up and see a DC-10 or a 747. The more you explore visual stimuli for their special features, the more meaningful your perception will be and the more you can use the information they provide.

Controlling Distorting Influences

When we process visual material, we are prone to distorting influences, which can cause us to make incorrect interpretations if we are not on guard against them. These influences are not caused by our perceptual habits, but by other factors.

Subliminal Cues

Often we become influenced by visual cues that are below our level of awareness. We take these cues in, but do not consciously register them along with the other cues we are noting. Advertisers and propagandists make use of this tendency in order to influence our perceptions about their products or causes. For example, suppose you are watching a movie about a person who makes a very favorable impression on you and in the course of this film that person smokes a particular brand of cigarette. Without your awareness, that brand can be perceived as belonging to the positive aura of the character, thereby deriving a halo of its own.

Irrelevant Cues

In similar fashion, perceptual interpretations can be influenced by cues of which we are aware, but which are nonetheless irrelevant. For instance, people often judge others more favorably if they see them clothed in designer fashions. They see the Gucci, Pucci, or Fiorucci label and make interpretations of the other person based on those labels. Labels are helpful in aiding our understanding of unfamiliar visual material, but labels, whether those of a designer or not, can also function to create misperceptions if we are not alert to that tendency. If we see a fish filet on a white porcelain platter garnished with thin lemon wedges and parsley we are apt to make different perceptual judgments than if that same fish filet is seen on a cracked plastic platter without the green and yellow flourishes. The fish will be perceived as fresher and more appetizing in the first situation than in the second.

Emotional Factors

How we feel and the biases we bring to bear have a great deal to do with our perceptual judgments. People tend to perceive things that are significant to them and not to see things that are unpleasant, thereby getting a distorted view of the world. In other words, we are inclined to see what we want to see and to misperceive what we do not want to see. In an experiment on visual perception, for example, a subject with prudish attitudes saw the word *whore* as *whole,* and in other ways distorted visual phenomena to make them more compatible with the self system.

Obliviousness to Influences

Underlying the factors cited is the most telling one of all, namely our tendency to be unaware that our perceptions are being influenced. In our belief that "what you see is what you get," we fool ourselves into thinking that there is a one-to-one correspondence between reality and the way we perceive the world. Knowing that your perceptions are your personal interpretations of what you see is a prime requisite of intelligent behavior.

PERCEPTUAL STYLE

Because perception is an interpretive process, it varies from individual to individual; everyone has a personal perceptual style. Perhaps you have seen the famous poster by Saul Steinberg depicting his map of the United States. Most of the map is taken up by New York City, although one or two other cities like Los Angeles manage to creep into the small space left between New York and the Pacific Ocean. The map is intended to be funny, but it does convey quite aptly many a New Yorker's perception of the country. Chances are a large number of Texans would draw a very different looking map, with Texas rather than New York as the hub of the United States. Both of these interpretations betray the same perceptual style, namely, an egocentric one in which the mapmaker sees the self as the center of the universe. Now let us look at some other perceptual styles.

Objective vs. Need-Oriented Styles

Although most people think they approach the world objectively, a person's values and needs often influence what is seen. Turning the old aphorism around, believing is seeing. One of the classic experiments proving the influence of needs in the perceptual process showed that children from impoverished backgrounds estimated the size of coins to be larger than did children of well-to-do backgrounds. Other needs besides materialistic ones can influence our perceptions. Another experiment revealed that people incorrectly estimated the length of rods when others in the group gave incorrect estimates. These subjects perceived the rods as they were described by the others, because of their need for acceptance. If you think you are immune from this process and make accurate judgments independent of your needs, try the following exercise.

Exercise

Get paper and pencil and write down a description of what an apple looks like in as much detail as you can, and then a description of what Richard M. Nixon looks like, in as much detail as you can.

Before checking your descriptions, look at the descriptions given by "E.R.":

An apple: Well, a delicious apple is usually bright red, shiny, hard and firm, and the shape is circular but wide at top and pointed at bottom with four or five bumps at the bottom. The color might not be completely red but green and red alternately, with white specks. At the top there is an indentation where the twig comes out. The twig is brown, sometimes leaves come off it.

Nixon: I can't describe him because I'm not into politics. Ugly, jowly. Ski slope nose, beady eyes, fat face, looks like a yucky

person, not nice clever, but yucky clever. Don't know what his
body looks like, only know his head. His hair is ugly, receding
hair line, balding.

The apple description is complete and quite objective. It de-
lineates the appearance of a specific apple variety and does not
generalize or offer a composite description of all apples. It is free
of value-laden phrases. It does include texture descriptions, which
were not called for, but these too are objective. The second
description, in contrast, mixes the visual with the attitudinal.
E.R. first states that she cannot describe Nixon because she is not
into politics, thus showing some awareness of her difficulty in
making perceptual judgments that stay true to the stimulus. But
then her description makes use of many value-laden adjectives
like *ugly, yucky,* and *not nice,* showing how E.R.'s feelings
about Nixon interfere with her ability to see him in a totally
objective way.

Now look at your descriptions. If you were able to complete
this exercise in an objective manner, fine. If you found that
your description was heavily influenced by your attitudes, try to
stay alert to this tendency whenever you make observations. Ask
yourself first, "What are my feelings and attitudes about this?"
Once identified, it will be easier to keep these feelings and
attitudes to the side while you are obtaining your visual data.

Global vs. Differentiated Styles

In dealing with visual material, some people tend to be more
absorbed with the total impression of the object or scene in front
of them; others tend to be absorbed with the impressions they
glean from the constituent parts. These two styles are known as
global and differentiated.

Developing a differentiated approach will generally enable
you to function more intelligently than a global approach. Differ-
entiators take in more of what they see. Global perceivers tend to
be swayed in their perceptual judgments by strong forces in the
visual field and miss details that could be important. No matter
which type of perceiver you tend to be, it will be helpful for you
to try the following exercises on a daily basis to improve your
differentiating ability.

Exercise

Whenever you meet someone new, or when you are sitting on a bus or train opposite someone, try to get a differentiated picture of that person. Scrutinize that person's appearance so that you can give an accurate description of such details as hair color, shape of hairline, eye color, shape of nose, shape of mouth, skin tone, contour of face, approximate height, type of body frame, and so on. This exercise is easy to do and, if you do it on a regular basis, it will train your differentiating ability in other situations as well.

Exercise

When you come across a photo in the newspaper or in a magazine, don't just glance at it and read the caption. Instead, look at it carefully and observe all the details. The caption will probably tell you who the people in the photo are, but ask yourself, what are the expressions on their faces, what are their body stances like, how are they clothed, where was this picture taken, what are the surroundings like? Not infrequently, people are swayed more by what is written in the caption than by what they see with their own eyes. A differentiator will sometimes learn more about what is going on by carefully observing the photograph than by reading the accompanying article. Not too long ago, for instance, a French newspaper ran a photo illustrating its article on El Salvador. An astute differentiator recognized that the photo was actually taken in Guatemala and proved that the news story was a hoax.

Flexible vs. Rigid Styles

The more unstructured the visual material is, the more these two styles come into play. Ambiguous visual material that lacks clarity or contains conflicting visual elements can be processed in a flexible or rigid manner, depending on your personal style.

You have probably heard of the Rorschach test, which consists of a series of inkblots designed by a Swiss psychiatrist, Hermann Rorschach, to interpret personality. People taking the test are asked to describe what they see in the blots. People with a flexible perceptual style can perceive a variety of forms within those blots, while those with a rigid style find it hard to see anything but ink blots. In general, it is helpful to develop flexibility in the way you look at visual material to leave yourself the possibility of interpreting it in different ways.

Exercise

Make up a set of your own blots by putting some dabs of ink or paint in the center of the page. Fold the page in half, ink side in, press the top surface but do not rub, as this will smudge the ink too much; open up and let dry. When your blot pictures are finished, use them to develop your flexibility in making perceptual interpretations. See how many different images you can make out in each blot. The possibilities are enormous and you want to try to take off any blinders you might be imposing on yourself. Remember, too, not just to focus on the whole blot, but practice your differentiating skills by looking for smaller percepts within the larger ones. This exercise is also good for practicing your skill with figure-ground reversals. If your inkblot has an enclosed white space, try to develop as many percepts as you can focusing on the white space as the figure and the ink as the ground.

Your tolerance for ambiguous visual material is related to your tolerance for material containing conflicting visual information. Do you notice conflicting elements or do you wash them out by seeing only what fits into your preconceptions? Jerome Bruner of Harvard performed an interesting experiment with students using a specially designed pack of playing cards. In this deck, some of the cards appeared in their natural state, but on others the colors were reversed. For example, a ten of hearts might be printed in black instead of red, and an ace of spades might be printed in red instead of black. In that way, Bruner introduced a conflict between color and form on some of his cards. When the cards were presented to students and they were asked to state what was being shown, Bruner found that many students had trouble seeing the alterations. Some dealt with the conflict by only responding to the color of the cards (calling a red ace of spades a heart, for example), some by only responding to the shape of the cards (calling a red ace of spades a black ace of spades), some by mixing the two colors (calling a red ace of spades a brown or purple ace of spades). Some students became confused by the altered cards and could not say what they had seen. Of course some were able to recognize the conflict and respond accordingly, calling a red ace of spades just that.

It is difficult to deal with material that conflicts with our expectations because we are used to seeing the world a certain way. The tendency to perceive the familiar and reject the unfamiliar is dramatically demonstrated by another experiment conducted with American and Mexican school teachers. Both groups were shown simultaneous images of a baseball player and a matador through a special optical device that exposed a different image to each eye. The Mexicans perceived only the matador and the Americans only the baseball player. To be able to see and act more intelligently, you have to be open to material that may be in conflict with what your past experience leads you to expect. Only when you keep yourself flexible can you really see what is going on around you.

IMPROVING YOUR VISION

There are several areas of vision in which people can usually benefit from practice: learning to shift focus more readily, expanding peripheral vision, taking in more detail, and tracking moving objects.

Shifting Focus

There is a tendency to keep fixating on an object when one is thinking about it. This is counterproductive, because your eyes register more information in the first moments of looking at something than when continuing to focus. Fixating can actually strain your eyes and interfere with good vision. It is better to consciously shift your gaze both to avoid fixating and to train yourself to take in more information. Wherever you are, make a conscious effort to move your eyes from place to place, from person to person. For example, as you walk down the street, keep your eyes shifting from object to object. Don't just look at the sidewalk or people in front of you but look at the stores, the trees, the cars at the curb, the sky between the buildings, and so on. Similarly, use your time sitting on the commuting train or bus by training your eyes to move from passenger to passenger. Try to shift your gaze every half-second. Do not look just at a person's face, but keep shifting your gaze to the chest, the arms, the torso, the legs, making sure to blink as your eyes shift focus. These exercises will not only increase your information handling capacity, but will rest your eyes at the same time.

Increasing Peripheral Vision

Although we are primarily aware of the sense impressions our eyes receive from objects directly in front of them, we also receive impressions from the periphery of the visual field. It is easy to test this for yourself. Pick up this book and hold it in front of you. With your gaze fixed straight ahead, slowly move the book to the side just until the point where you can no longer make out the book. Now wave the book. Although you cannot see the book, you are aware of something moving in the periphery. Try another experiment. Make a fist and hold it in front of you. While looking straight ahead, slowly move your fist to the side of your visual field to the point where it is not visible and then move it back to the point where you can just make it out. Now uncurl your fingers one at a time and try to see all five of them. Chances are you cannot see them as separate digits. These two experiments demonstrate that your brain makes very little use of the information coming to it from the periphery of the visual field. Being able to use your peripheral vision expands your brain's capacity and increases your ability to respond intelligently.

You can enhance your peripheral vision through the following exercises. These exercises are tiring, so we suggest limiting yourself to no more than fifteen-minute sessions and stopping earlier if you feel too much strain. To do the exercises, sit in a comfortable chair facing a blank wall space with a fixation point marked on it at the level of your eyes. You will be keeping your eyes focused on this point, but you should blink frequently to lessen eye fatigue. The blinking will have the same effect as eye-shifting in reducing strain.

Exercise

As you gaze in front of you, concentrate on the impressions coming to you from the sides. Try to make out the discrete objects in the blur. At first you will probably see nothing, but as you repeat this exercise over several days, you will find that your peripheral vision becomes sharper.

Exercise

Using 8½-by-11 inch paper, draw a letter of the alphabet and/or a digit from 0 to 9 on each sheet, using the full length of the paper. Color in the letters or digits with bright ink or crayon so that they are highly visible. Shuffle the papers so you can't anticipate the sequence. Place the papers on a table within your reach, but outside of your visual field when you are sitting in your practice chair. Pick up the papers one by one and try to read the letters on them.

As you become better at these exercises, your peripheral identifications will come more quickly. As that happens, enlarge the angle at which you present material to your eyes, eventually up to seventy to eighty degrees, which is the range of outer limit. Once you can perform the two exercises at an angle of about seventy degrees, you are ready to continue with Exercise 3, using smaller and more intricate objects.

Exercise _____

Prepare another set of alphabet cards, reducing the size of the letters by a third, and practice as before. After that, continue with another set of cards of still smaller letters, and so on until you find you are able to make out letters that are quite small. Eventually you may find that you can even read a large-type book in the peripheral area.

_____

It is, of course, more sensible for you to read in your direct line of vision, as your vision there will always be better. Nevertheless, by training your eyes to take in more information from the sides, you keep yourself more alert and start to use brain pathways that otherwise would be dormant. When peripheral vision is not developed fully, it not only keeps your neural pathways unexercised, but makes it easier for them to decay. These exercises are vital to your brain health, as well as providing a source of additional information to use.

Taking in More Detail

Aside from the usual loss of detail in peripheral vision, we also tend to miss detail even when objects are placed directly in front of our eyes. How often have you been asked to describe a certain person or object and found yourself answering, "I didn't notice"? To get into the habit of noticing more detail under ordinary visual circumstances, try the following exercise and do it at least once or twice each day for about a minute.

Exercise _____

Pick up any object within your reach, hold it in your hand, and look at it carefully. Turn it around, look at it from different angles until you are sure you have taken it all in. While you are looking at it, really concentrate on seeing what it is like. Suppose you picked up a pencil. Describe it to yourself: How long is it, what color is it painted, how many separate flat sides are there comprising the surface of the pencil, what is imprinted on it, what color is the imprinting, how is the eraser attached to the wooden shaft, by metal or plastic? What shade of metal is it? What kind of design is stamped onto the metal, what is the shape of the eraser, how rounded is it? And so on. You will be amazed at the different aspects there are to a pencil, which you have never noticed before. The experience with the pencil can be repeated with every object you pick up.

Another way to improve your ability to take in more detail is to speed up the rate at which you absorb visual material. You can practice by enlisting a friend to help you.

Exercise

Buy a set of flash cards that have words or sums printed on them, or make your own flash cards depicting simple objects or words. Have a friend flash these cards in front of you, allowing no more viewing time than the actual flashing movement of the hand requires. While initially you probably will not be able to make anything out, after a time you will find that you can begin to recognize the material on the cards with greater and greater ease.

Tracking Moving Objects

A lot of people have difficulty tracking moving objects, a phenomenon that becomes apparent at a baseball stadium. Many times spectators can only tell by the movement of the players where the ball has gone, because they lose sight of the ball itself. If you have trouble tracking moving objects, there are various exercises you can try. Watching the neighborhood kids play baseball is an excellent exercise. Keep your eyes on the ball rather than the players. Another simple exercise to do on the street is reading license plates of moving cars. For more serious work on tracking at home, try the following exercise.

Exercise

For this exercise you need a record player or turntable that is at a comfortable viewing height. Put on a record and try to read the label as the turntable is revolving. If this is too hard to do, which it probably will be at first, start by making your own discs out of large-size index cards, or paper of similar thickness. Simply cut out rounds, with a hole in the middle for the turntable spindle, and print various messages on the cards in large, bold letters. Prepare a variety of cards and shuffle the order so that you will not know beforehand what is imprinted on the disc. Then put each one on the turntable and try to read the message. You may want to start at a slow speed first, and later increase the speed at which you try tracking the message.

USING ALL YOUR SENSES

Though vision is your most highly developed sense, the others are important and should not be underestimated or underused. Just as your visual perception can be improved, you can do a lot to increase the efficiency of your other primary perceptual modes. For intelligent functioning, you must develop all your perceptual possibilities, not just to clue you in to what is going on around you, but to make use of neural pathways that otherwise lie dormant and start to deteriorate.

Hearing

We tend to be careless listeners, tuning in to sound only when someone speaks to us or when we are listening to a specific source, such as the radio, a speaker at a lecture, or musicians at a concert. Sound, however, is around us constantly telling us about our environment, if only we listen. The following exercises will help you improve your aural perception and enable you to make better use of the information coming to you through your ears.

Exercise

For one minute each day, stop what you are doing, and just listen to the sounds around you. You will be surprised at what you hear that ordinarily you are oblivious to. It may be that you suddenly notice through sound that a dog is on the street, a bird is on the window ledge, a car is approaching, or heat is coming through the radiator. Sound provides many clues about what is going on around you if you train yourself to use the information that is available for you to hear.

Exercise

The next time you are in a new environment, close your eyes for just sixty seconds, and concentrate on the sounds you hear. Suppose you are in the reception room of a company to which you are applying for a job. Do you hear people's voices? Are they laughing, even-toned, shouting? Does it sound like a pleasant, active, calm, or erratic working environment? Are there people coming and going in the reception room? What are the sounds of their gait and what do those sounds reveal? Do the footsteps stop near the area of the reception desk (fellow applicants) or pass beyond (employees)? With just one minute of listening you will be able to learn a lot about the company's atmosphere that will enrich the picture you ordinarily take in only with your eyes.

Incidentally, you can expand this exercise to include your other nonvisual senses. What does the texture of the chair covering you're sitting on feel like? What does the place smell like? What is the tactile quality of your interviewer's handshake?

Adapt this exercise to any new situation you encounter—a visit to a new friend's apartment, a tour of an unfamiliar town, a trip to the beach, and so on. Try to find out about the new environment by the sounds that are essential to it.

Because we live in an age of electronic amplification, our hearing is becoming less acute. The very high volume sounds of the rock concert have been known to damage people's hearing permanently. Similarly the noise pollution of heavy machinery, jet planes, traffic, and your neighbor's stereo tends to accustom you to louder and louder sounds, making it more difficult for you to perceive auditory information coming to you at lower volume levels.

Exercise

This exercise is designed to improve your auditory acuity for low-level sound and to provide a needed rest from overly loud sound. Whenever you listen to your TV or stereo set, turn down the volume to at least one-quarter of the volume to which you are accustomed. At this level you will still be able to hear the sound comfortably. After you have been listening for a while at the lower volume, turn it down still further to the point where you have to strain somewhat to make out the sound. Keep listening at this level for as long as you can without experiencing discomfort and without losing out on something important that you want to hear. Then turn the volume up, but only slightly, to eliminate strain, and still keep it below your usual volume level. Within two weeks you probably will find that the comfortable sound level for you is much lower than it used to be and that your auditory acuity has improved.

This exercise can also be modified to use in conversations at home. When you are talking at the dinner table or on the phone, consciously try to speak at a lower volume and ask the others to do the same. People tend to adjust their speaking voices to the sound level around them and speak unnecessarily loudly because they are accustomed to such high noise levels on the streets, in the movies, and practically everywhere else they go.

Exercise

To develop your ability to break sound down into its component parts, start by listening to music. Use your favorite type of music, beginning with small ensembles and working your way up to orchestral music. As you listen, try to follow only one of the instruments rather than the total sound. Become aware of the musical line being followed by the instrument you have selected, whether it is the violin or clarinet, so that you become familiar enough with it to sing that part. The difficulty of this exercise will depend on how much musical training you have had and how much you are used to listening to music. Do not be discouraged if you cannot reproduce the part of your instrument: it often is possible to do so only after considerable training.

You can increase the complexity of this exercise by learning to track a second instrument in the same piece of music. Once you have the second instrument clear, relisten, but this time try to track both instruments at once. This may sound absolutely impossible to you at first, but remember that symphonic conductors can listen to the diverse musical elements of the complete orchestra at one time, and they have the same ear design as you do. The only difference is that they have had years of training to differentiate instrumental sounds, whereas you are just a beginner. Developing hearing skill takes as much practice as running a marathon, but it can be done.

Another variation on this exercise is to practice tracking two voices at once. This exercise is most conveniently done if you have two recorders available, and tapes of two different people talking. All you do is play them both at once and try to follow the two voices at one time. Depending on what type of equipment you have at home you can vary this procedure: listen to a radio talk show and play a recorded tape at the same time; or plug in two radios and listen to two talk shows, or listen to your radio and TV with the picture turned off; or use a record player with a disc of recorded poetry or drama overlaid on a radio talk show.

Without training, most people can follow only one conversation at a time, but with repeated practice you should be able to make sense out of two simultaneous conversations, even if you do not hear them both completely. Some people have been able to track three conversations at once, given a lot of practice. Developing this ability has obvious benefits in that it keeps you more alert to what is going on around you in a lot of important situations: business meetings committee conferences, social affairs, and so on. You will be able to track speaking voices much better, however, even if you only practice tracking musical instruments. The process is the same—you train your brain to process more of the aural information that is out there.

Smelling

Although odors abound all around you, you probably perceive very little with your nose because you are not used to integrating this information with that coming to you through other channels. Your nose, however, can tell you a lot that your other perceptual modes, including vision, cannot, because smell lingers on. Our children, who are used to processing information received through the nose, often knew what we were about in their absence. When they came home in the evening, they could tell if we had had visitors, and often who the visitors were. They were aware of how each of our close friends smelled—identifying them by their usual toiletries and/or idiosyncratic body odors, which still wafted in the air. If we had been out for the evening, they could also tell a great deal about where we had been. They picked up the cigarette smoke on our clothing, the cooking odors from the restaurant, the smell of the park if we had walked by the river. We doubt that our children are uniquely gifted in this way. Rather, they have learned to interpret the sensory information their noses provide, and so can you. In societies more dependent on smell than ours, it is perfectly natural for people to have acute olfactory perceptions. In hunting societies, it is an everyday occurrence to track down animals by the odor trail they leave behind. These people differentiate the smells in the woods better than we can differentiate between two perfumes. Our olfactory perceptions are so poorly utilized that we even have to rely on smoke detectors when we are sleeping to know when our house is burning. Your nose is the best smoke detector there is, if you would only use it more. You can train yourself to process olfactory information that you currently ignore, so that you keep more in tune with what is happening around you. Below are some simple exercises to improve your olfactory acuity.

Exercise

Take a minute each day to concentrate on the smells in your environment. Walk around the room you happen to be in. What can you smell? Are there the smells of other people—traces left behind from a cigarette, a cologne, body perspiration? What odors can you detect from nearby? Is an aroma coming in from the kitchen, or from the restaurant downstairs? Is there any odor from traffic exhaust coming in through the window? What about the objects surrounding you? How does the book in front of you smell? Pick it up and smell it. Does it smell musty; does it smell as if it had been handled by others; does it smell like fresh paper and ink? Don't forget to smell yourself too. Lift your hands to your nose. What do they smell like? Can you smell what you have been touching with your hands? How about your general body scent? How can you describe it? One minute of active, concentrated smelling every day will make you much more sensitive to odors even when you are not consciously working on it.

Exercise

The purpose of this exercise is to make you aware of the special smells associated with a particular place. You can probably give a good visual description of your home, your place of work, your favorite section of town, but could you tell somebody what each of these places smells like? Each time you visit any location, try to construct a smell-picture of that spot and put it into words so that someone else would be able to identify it from your description. Every place has its own odor and you can learn to know where you are just by smell alone.

Exercise

Another helpful exercise is learning to differentiate among similar smells. You can practice this in several different ways. A simple method is using your spice rack. Blindfold yourself and have an assistant hand you the jars or boxes one at a time for you to identify by aroma only. By reversing roles, you can help your assistant become a more acute olfactory perceiver as well. Another method is to have your assistant walk you through the local botanical gardens blindfolded, while you try to identify the flowers from their aroma. You can also try this exercise at the perfume counter or at the soap shelf in a store.

In doing the exercises to increase your olfactory sensitivity, there are a few things to keep in mind. Obviously, if you have a cold and your nose is stuffed, that is not a good time to practice. When your nose is too dry, sensitivity is reduced, since the olfactory membrane should be moist to pick up odors. If you have a hard time discriminating odors, it could be related to the shape of your nasal passage, which sometimes blocks the passage of odor-laden air into the nasal clefts. In this case, you just have to sniff hard. Try to practice the exercises in the late morning or late afternoon, which are the times of day when you have the most sensitivity to odor. Your sensitivity is markedly decreased after lunch, but if you do not eat lunch, sensitivity will remain high from the late morning through to late afternoon. People with dark pigmentation are more sensitive to smell than light-pigmented persons because the pigmentation of the olfactory membrane acts to absorb more odor, just as dark clothes absorb more light. If you are very fair, you may have a more difficult time developing your olfactory sensitivity, but then you just have to try harder. Children also have a harder time at smelling than do adults, because their olfactory membranes are less pigmented. When you do the exercises for smell perception, do not smell one object too long. The olfactory membranes can suffer from fatigue and cease to register a scent after a certain point. You need a break in between so that the receptors can revive. Breathing out through the nose will also restore your smelling efficiency.

Tasting

In this era of gourmet cooks and international cuisine we tend to think of ourselves as pretty sophisticated when it comes to taste. Many of us no longer have to rely on tea-tasters or wine tasters to know a good drink from a bad one. But the very fact that professional tasters exist indicates that we have the potential for finer taste perceptions than most of us put to use. We're not going to suggest that you eat more, but that you become more aware of the taste of the things you eat and that you increase the variety of the tastes that you sample.

The perception of taste resides much more in your nervous system than in what you eat. We have receptors for four basic tastes: sweet, sour, bitter, and salt, and what we end up tasting depends on which receptors are activated. We can taste bitterness at much lower concentrations than we notice the other three tastes, probably a built-in warning system against poisonous substances. Often we have better perception of saltiness when our sweet receptors are activated at the same time. This is how the custom developed of putting salt on melon or jelly on a salted cracker. As with smell, your sense of taste can become fatigued from overstimulation. That is why a piece of candy in your mouth seems tasteless after a while unless you roll it over. This puts it in contact with other tastebuds, which are not fatigued and which can therefore send taste messages to your brain. To develop your sense of taste, try the following exercises.

Exercise

The next time you eat, when you take your first bite, make it a very small one and concentrate on the taste. Chew, suck, or savor the bite very slowly, with your eyes closed, giving the taste of the food your full attention. You will find that this not only helps you enjoy your food more and cuts down on the amount you eat, but it will also develop your ability to differentiate among different tastes.

Exercise

Whenever you eat out, at a friend's house or at a restaurant, make it a habit to try to figure out the recipe. See if you can taste the component ingredients and flavors. Check out your perceptions with the chef so that you can correct any misperceptions you might have.

Although the way something tastes to you will not necessarily correspond to the way it tastes to somebody else, you can still increase your own sensitivity and ability to discriminate among the various taste sensations that come your way. Taste probably evolved as a protective mechanism to direct us to beneficial foods and steer us away from harmful ones. Don't let your taste become merely a gourmet guide, but use your taste perceptions to know your world better.

Touching

Our touch perceptions are an important way of processing information that is essential to our well-being, but touch has been in disrepute for a long time, only recently coming back into fashion. Though we have been told to "keep your hands to yourself," the basic nature of touch as a means of knowing the world is evident in the way we speak: "He is very touchy about that"; "He rubs me the wrong way"; "Don't forget to get in touch with me." We usually only touch things that we have to handle, and thereby deprive ourselves of touch perceptions of other objects, relying instead on visual impressions. As a result, our touch perceptions lose acuity and many of us would find it hard to differentiate objects by touch alone, unless there are gross disparities between them. It is a good idea to practice your touch perceptions as well as your other perceptual modes.

Exercise

Spend sixty seconds each day touching an object. With your eyes closed, concentrate on the tactile sensations. Pass the object from hand to hand, making sure you experience it from all its sides, around all its contours, over all its surfaces, into all its crevices. Note the sensation of the texture on your skin—is it rough, smooth, tingly, tickly? How can you describe it so that someone else could pick up that object and know what you meant?

People who are not sighted are much more capable of knowing objects through touch perception than are those with vision. Some persons, sighted and unsighted, have been trained to perceive colors and read letters through touch alone. This merely indicates that you have a long way to go in developing your own tactile sensitivity.

Synthesizing

We have been talking about different perceptual modes as if they were separate domains. Actually, your perceptions from one modality are connected to perceptions from other modalities. In the exercises, we tried to isolate these perceptual systems artificially, by having you close your eyes in order to smell or touch, for example, but in the ordinary course of events your perceptions are enhanced by the ability of your different perceptual systems to work together. Probably you have discovered that you can taste your food better when you can smell it too and that you do not enjoy eating when you have a cold as much as you do when your nasal passages are clear. This is because vapors from food stimulate the olfactory receptors as you start to eat, giving you enhanced perception. Similarly, the odors passing through the nostrils can travel to the taste receptors in the mouth, stimulating your appetite by the mere smell and actually giving you a foretaste of the food. Just as taste and smell enhance each other, so do the other modalities interact. A flower is perceptually enhanced when we can smell it as we look at it; food is perceptually enhanced if we can hear the sizzle of the frying pan as well as smell the aroma wafting up from the food. Try to take in objects and experiences using as many perceptual avenues as possible. The exercises are meant to train you in using those perceptual abilities that are ordinarily underutilized, but they are no substitute for getting to process information through as wide a spectrum of perceptual modes as possible.

Perceptual systems not only enhance each other; they also can substitute for each other in a curious way. In a process called *synesthesia,* stimulation of one sensory system can create perceptions in another system. You have probably experienced something close to this if you ever had a blow to the eye: the pressure on the eye is perceived as light, resulting in the experience of "seeing stars." In true synesthesia, however, the perceptual experience occurs without any stimulation of the corresponding sense organ. Musicians with true pitch, for example, are frequently able to "see" the various tones as having characteristic colors. Others report "tasting" certain visual scenes, and some persons "hear" tones when they look at certain colors.

Research suggests that everyone is born with the capacity for synesthesia, but that we subdue and eventually obliterate that capacity as we grow older. One of the appeals of mind-expanding drugs such as LSD has been that they expand the boundaries of perception and make possible the experience of synesthesia. You can try developing your synesthetic capacities without drugs, however, by use of the meditation techniques discussed more fully in the chapter "Hidden Powers of the Mind." Because the sensory receptors tend to become fatigued with continual stimulation, meditation and relaxation techniques serve to rest and rejuvenate these receptors, making it possible to perceive more vividly and for perceptual crossovers to occur. Although you may not see the practicality of developing synesthesia, the benefits are not just esoteric. In addition to the ecstasy that people feel when having synesthetic experiences, it is a way to know the world more fully. At present, we tend to perceive things in a one-dimensional way; we either see, hear, or smell them. Occasionally we see, smell, and touch all at once. But how many of us know the color of sounds? By developing a richer perceptual capability we can not only remember things better because they become more vivid, but we can begin to understand and grasp things in an entirely different way.

THE OTHER SENSES

Because we are used to thinking in terms of the five primary senses, we tend to remain unaware that our sensory potential is much greater. Our total number of senses is still unknown, but current estimates are that they come closer to twenty than five. Just for starters, we have sensors that monitor our body functions such as blood sugar detectors, mouth dryness detectors, and bladder-distension detectors. Our sense of touch can be broken down into receptors for heat, for cold, for pressure, for position, for change of stimulation, and so on. We also have a sense of verticality and a sense of balance. Despite this impressive list and our ability to integrate these different sensations into higher order patterns, what we know of the world is very limited compared to what could be known and even what is known by less complex organisms. We speak about the narrowness of a bird's eye view, but a human's eye view is just as limited. What we perceive of the world is in part restricted by our sensory equipment, and in part by our hypotheses about the world, which determine what we expect to perceive. We favor what is most useful for us and ignore the rest, assuming that our perceptions represent the world exactly as it is. We may think it is a quiet, peaceful day but elephants, horses, and other animals can feel the tremblings of an incipient earthquake. We may see the sun standing still over our heads at noon, but the rabbit sees its slow movement in the sky. Other animals perceive the direction of a magnetic field, or the change from tap water to distilled water, or ultraviolet light, or the polarization of light, and so on. In short, our perceptions add up to only a fraction of what is out there. We have to be careful not to presume that what we see is what there is. We think that seeing is believing, but function as if believing is seeing.

Your perceptions will remain limited if you take for granted that what you see tells you the whole story. What you see is only a workable hypothesis about the nature of the world. It comes in very handy, but it can also lead you astray. Many so-called extra-sensory perceptions are really sensory experiences that most of us have programmed ourselves not to have because they do not fit in with our preconceptions. Once you stop predefining what the world is like, you will be able to perceive more of it.

IMPROVING MEMORY

Your memory, just like most other people's, is working far below its maximum capacity. How often have you been unable to recall a name, a date, or fact, even though you were sure that the information was lurking somewhere in your head? Probably you've also had the experience of unexpectedly remembering something you thought you had completely forgotten. You are not alone. Research has demonstrated that we have a vast storehouse of memories that is usually not available for our immediate use. Recent investigations have shown that, through electric stimulation of the brain, people have been able to recall events and material that seemed to have been lost. Under hypnosis others are able to remember many details that were lost to them in a conscious state. Reports from persons who were sure they were going to die or who were momentarily clinically dead also make clear how much is stored away in memory of which we are ordinarily unaware. These persons typically report going through a life review process in which all the important events of their lives, many presumed forgotten, flash by in a moment. On a less dramatic plane, you probably have had dreams in which you dealt with memories that you were unaware of while awake. It appears that once a memory trace is established, it is there for good; you just have to learn how to activate it. This can be accomplished by familiarizing yourself with the memory process and how it works. The difference between you and the memory experts you read about—quiz-show contestants with all the answers, performers who can remember everyone in the audience by name, people with photographic memory—is that they know how to convert new information into memory traces and how to activate those stored memories. Because of their skill, they can also put a lot more memories into storage. You can develop those skills too.

WHY RELY ON YOUR MEMORY?

You may be wondering why, if people are capable of total recall, so few people have good memories. Memory failure is largely a modern phenomenon. In earlier societies memory was actively cultivated. Holy men of India, for example, devoted themselves to memorizing volumes of the sacred writings. Similarly, the ancient Greek and Roman orators commonly committed speeches of several hours' length to memory. The oral tradition of memorizing material for transmission to others was a necessity before the printing press and inexpensive paper were available. Once you have books, pencils, and pads, you no longer have to remember as much. That is why classical memory-training became obsolete during the Renaissance, with the development of the printing press and availability of books. Today we do not want to take the time to commit information to memory that we can easily look up in the encyclopedia, dictionary, or almanac. Such personal facts as names, addresses, phone numbers, and appointments are jotted down in a diary that conveniently relieves us from having to remember today's date or the events to follow in the coming weeks. In countries where books and writing materials are harder to come by, people tend to have better memories. Educational researchers coming back from China, where textbooks are in short supply, have reported that the children there are capable of committing huge amounts of material to memory. A child will not only know his or her own lines in a play, but be able to recite the entire play. Similarly, children in China who have to share a book will remember the text so they can take the book home in their minds.

The more you use your memory, the better it becomes. Some people have the notion that they will clutter up their minds if they try to remember a lot of material, but the reverse is what actually happens. There is no limit to the amount of material you can store; the more you have already put away, the simpler it is to add to your memory bank. Old memories facilitate new memories and make them easier to file and retrieve. If you are worried about overtaxing your memory, it might help you to know that even without trying you will probably store more than one quadrillion bits of information in your lifetime. Much of the time you are not even aware of the fact that you are using your memory. Just by reading this page, for example, you are activating all sorts of memory traces: the shapes of the letters of the alphabet, the sounds they represent, and the meanings of the words they form. Now you take these memories for granted just as you do memories for the names and faces of your friends, the route home from the bus stop, the way to tie your shoelace, and so on. These memories become automatic because they involve basic principles to be discussed later on. For the time being we just want to emphasize how much you use your memory and that it is easy to do so when memories are properly stored.

Despite the fact that you can't overtax your memory, too many meaningless bits of remembered information can be taxing on your equanimity. You could, like the memory experts, train yourself to remember all sorts of data—lists of dates, telephone numbers, statistics, or international train schedules—but there is very little reason, other than theatrical, to spend the time and effort memorizing this type of information, and there are good reasons why you should not. Take, for example, the case of a Russian newspaper reporter who was studied for a thirty-year period by Alexander Luria, the Russian psychologist. The journalist had no apparent limit to his memory capacity. He could remember lists of numbers, nonsense syllables, complex mathematical formulas, or anything else you put before him and he could remember this material correctly years afterward. He committed to memory a list of several hundred repetitive non-sense syllables and was able to reproduce the list eight years later without error. His technique for remembering this material was to use visual images. While he had no problem remembering things, he was bothered by his inability to forget. He found him-self being swamped with mental images that he had difficulty brushing aside. He had to develop a technique for forgetting and making his images disappear. Unless you want to make a career out of your memory ability, it is better to use your memory consciously only for material that is meaningful to you. We are inundated by information, much of which we need, but much of which we do not need. In part, our tendency to forget is a way of protecting ourselves from that mass of data already deposited in the memory bank. Since it is not useful, we leave it lying dormant. Don't waste your time memorizing irrelevant infor-mation, but do make use of the techniques outlined here to remember everything that is important to you.

HOW YOUR MEMORY WORKS

There are three stages in the memory system: immediate mem-ory, short-term memory, and long-term memory. Each system has a different purpose and it is important that you learn to use each as effectively as possible. Sometimes you might only want to use your immediate memory, sometimes you may want to stop at the short-term memory stage. But if you want information to be remembered for more than a minute, it must pass through all three stages.

Your immediate memory lets you remember something just long enough to respond to it. This system registers the information coming to you through your sense organs; it appears as an image that lasts for less than a second. The immediate memory system (or sensory register) can hold this image only momentarily because the image must give way to new sensory stimuli coming in. You have a sensory register for visual and auditory information, as well as for the other sense modalities. Although the images are a literal record of what you have seen or heard, they last only briefly and are lost unless you process them through your short- and long-term memory systems. As you walk down a street, for example, various images reach your eyes and ears: you see the traffic light, the cars parked at the curb, the pedestrians coming your way, and you hear the horn beep, the brakes screech, the people talking. All these sensory images enter your immediate memory but are lost in a second if you do not do something to make them stick. Usually there is no reason to retain these images and you let them pass in and out of your awareness. If your attention should be caught by any particular image, however—a pedestrian falling, a car going over a curb—that image passes from the sensory register into the short-term memory system.

Let's take a closer look at how these two systems operate in another typical setting. Suppose you want to place a person-to-person call. You phone the operator and request the number. The operator hears the number and keeps it in her or his immediate memory just long enough to dial it for you. After that the operator's sensory register is clear to receive the other numbers that will be pouring in. You have to remember the number for a longer time than the operator does. You have to look it up in your phone book and have it in your mind while dialing the operator and waiting for the operator to answer your call. Your immediate memory is too short-lived for this process and the image would decay unless you did something to keep the memory alive. By focusing your attention on the phone number and, perhaps, repeating it over and over to yourself (rehearsal), the image passes from your immediate memory into your short-term memory system.

In these two examples you can see that attention is the key factor that determines what goes into your short-term memory system. Unless you give incoming information your attention, it will not enter your short-term memory and be available later. More people suffer from insufficient attention than from loss of memory. Information literally passes them by unless they make some effort at the first stage in the memory process to grasp onto the sensory image. Your short-term memory system only starts to work after you consciously direct your attention to incoming information and sort it out as something important to remember. Even so, short-term memory is very limited.

Ordinarily, your short-term memory can retain information for half a minute at the most. (That's almost thirty times longer than your immediate memory, but a short time, nonetheless.) In addition, your short-term memory is also limited in the number of items it can retain at one time. For most people the magic number is seven, give or take two. Trying to remember more than seven items at any one time can interfere with your ability to retain even the basic seven. You can get around this, however, by grouping the material you want to remember. Basically what this means is that you organize new information into seven chunks rather than keeping it in discrete bits and pieces. The telephone company uses this principle in making up local phone numbers: they are never more than seven digits long, and even so are divided into two chunks to help you remember them. A phone number is not listed as 6-6-3-1-5-1-4, which would tax you at the upper limit of seven pieces, but as 663-1514, to reduce the number to two chunks that are easier to retain. Now that phone numbers are more complex with the addition of area codes, the phone companies group the numbers for you into three chunks so you can remember them. Overloading your short-term memory by working with more than seven chunks at any time can easily cause you to forget everything.

If short-term memory holds information only for half a minute, how do you ever get to remember anything for an extended period of time? As long as you actively direct your attention to information in your short-term memory system, you can keep it alive indefinitely. Attention determines what goes into short-term memory and it also determines how long it stays in your short-term memory.

While you are repeating and rehearsing information in the short-term memory, it becomes associated with information already in your long-term memory system, and the two connect. As this happens, the information is transferred from the short-term into the long-term memory system, where it remains indefinitely. Apparently, as the transfer is being effected, the brain goes through corresponding chemical processes that mark this transfer. These changes, involving protein synthesis, depend very heavily on your biochemical balance, which we will discuss in the chapter "The Care and Feeding of Your Brain."

After information enters your long-term memory system, it goes through several periods of consolidation—one in the first ten minutes after exposure, one during the first night's sleep after exposure, and one period some time during the next two weeks. Because of this, it is helpful to have short reviews of the new material. Two weeks after storing new information, it no longer has to be rehearsed but can stay alive even without active attention on your part. In contrast to the short-term memory, there are no limits on the amount of items your long-term memory can hold. In fact, the more information you have stored, the easier it is to add on to, because the possibilities for richer associations and better integration of the new material are increased.

You are probably wondering why, if your memories are all alive and well in the long-term memory system, you can't remember half the things you want to. The problem is that we have trouble retrieving the stored information. It is all there, but we do not know how to get it out. Sometimes you are aware of this, as when you have something on the tip of your tongue, as the saying goes. You *know* you know but you just can't get hold of it. At other times you feel as if you have lost the information completely. In both instances the information is there, although seemingly inaccessible to you. The secret to being able to get information out of your memory closet more easily is to put it away right in the first place. If you throw things haphazardly into your clothes closet, you can never find what you want when you need it. Similarly, your memories will be hard to find if they are not neatly put away.

As we have indicated so far, three key factors in improving your memory are attention, grouping, and organization. First, you consciously have to attend to information so it can pass from your immediate memory into short-term memory. Second, you have to chunk information so you will be able to retain more than the usual seven bits of data in your short-term memory.

Third, you have to organize the new information by developing strong associations between it and stored material in the long-term memory system. Let's cover these three factors now in more detail.

Attention

The degree to which you attend to any information is determined in part by the information and in part by you. Certain things have more attention-getting value than others; they catch your notice without any effort on your part. When our immediate memory system receives sensory images that are unusual, we automatically pay attention. Bright colors, sudden noises, a change in pattern and other novel or distinctive stimuli command our attention and have a better chance of passing into our short-term memory systems. Thus, the road engineer uses flashing lights to warn us away, as does the movie house to draw us in. Advertisers will try to catch you with a brightly colored ad, and a textbook publisher might print important words in red rather than black to make them stand out and become more memorable. Your attention is grabbed every day in this way, but let's see it at work right now.

Exercise _____

Read through the following list of words and then turn the page and complete the exercise as directed on the bottom of page 87.

wind	dog	string	house	bone	sleep
yard	fish	dish	pear	nose	door
jar	desk	Australia	leaf	pig	stick
life	death	song	car	toy	book
screwdriver	tent	ear	cat	ball	lake

See page 87 for the instructions for completing this exercise.

Once you have finished the exercise, look at what you have written down. Chances are, you did not remember more than seven of the words in the list, if that many, but which ones did you remember? Most people remember the word *Australia* because it stands out from the others. It is unique because it is the only place name, and only proper noun with a capital letter. *Screwdriver* similarly tends to be remembered as the only other polysyllabic word besides *Australia*. Some people find it easy to remember the words *fish* and *dish*. This pair of words has attention-getting value because it rhymes and therefore is catchy as well as distinctive. For similar reasons *life* and *death* tend to be remembered. These words stand out from the rest by forming a meaningful pair. Perhaps you remembered the words *wind* and *lake*. These two words are not particularly distinctive in and of themselves, but they are attention-getters because of their place in the list—namely, first and last. This is known as the *primacy-recency effect*.

While certain things will attract your attention more than others, you can also consciously direct your attention to information that you want to remember. Often, different stimuli compete for your attention; because it is hard to concentrate on more than one at a time, you must focus attention on the material that is most important to you. Focusing attention sounds easier than it is. Not only do you have to make a conscious decision to focus, but you must try to screen out all other incoming stimuli at the same time. Because many stimuli have a strong demand quality and because we are by nature curious, it is hard to shut ourselves off from what is going on around us. So, if you want to remember particular material, follow these steps to improve your attention:

1. Make a conscious decision that you want to remember a given piece of information;

2. Remind yourself that you are going to focus on that piece of information and only on that;

3. Set yourself a definite time span, to make the focusing job easier for you;

4. Remove yourself to a place where there will be a minimum of distracting stimuli;

5. Shut out as many extraneous stimuli as possible. Use a white sound machine to cover conversational sounds, sit with your back to the window so there is less temptation to look out and see what is going on, pick a time of day when there are not apt to be competing activities to draw your attention away.

6. Divide your focusing time into short periods with breaks in between.

Exercise from page 86: Take paper and pencil and write down as many words as you can remember from the list. When you are done, go back to page 86 to analyze your responses.

Another important aid in focusing your attention is the way you structure the time you spend at this activity. Before, we mentioned the primacy-recency effect; the tendency to attend more to the first and last items that you come across. You can't, of course, dictate to the information you are trying to remember what should come first and what should come last, but you can introduce more first and last points. When you want to focus attention on certain material, divide it into smaller blocks, with breaks in between. To illustrate, if you were to do the previous exercise as five separate exercises (1 per line), you would have five opportunities to experience primacy and recency effects, rather than one.

Grouping and Organization

Grouping information into chunks enables you to keep more than seven bits of information in your short-term memory at one time. Some material, like phone numbers, comes already grouped, but most of the time you will have to do the grouping. Suppose you are presented with a list of numbers you have to remember:

0 9 1 8 2 7 3 6 4 5

Since there are ten digits in this series, chances are you will find it impossible to remember all of them, even for immediate repetition. Try it out. Get yourself a piece of paper and pencil, read through all the numbers, then write down the list. Or, ask a friend to read off the numbers and repeat the numbers back. After you try remembering the list as ten separate digits, make the list easier to remember by grouping it into sets of three digits each:

091 827 364 5

Now if you test yourself again, you will find the list easier either to write down or repeat back to your friend. Even though chunking is efficient, you probably will not be able to remember this list for more than a minute. If you want to retain it longer, then you need more than chunking. You need to make the list meaningful by identifying some principle by which the numbers can be grouped. Look carefully at the list and you will notice that it includes all the single digits, starting with zero, in pairs from lowest to highest, from next lowest to next highest, and so on: from 0 to 9, from 1 to 8, from 2 to 7, from 3 to 6, from 4 to 5. Now you don't have to remember the individual numbers any more or four groups of meaningless numbers; you can remember one principle. If you want to remember the individual numbers and do not need to remember their particular order in the list, it is even easier to remember that the list contains all the numbers from 0 to 9, and nothing else. In this form you will be able to remember the numbers in the list forever. In short, when you want to commit material to memory, if you make it meaningful you will be able to store it away in your long-term memory indefinitely.

We know that you usually don't have to go around remembering lists of numbers. But you often do have to remember series of items that are also seemingly meaningless. Take your shopping list, for instance. Perhaps you have written one down—a good idea—but you have forgotten to take it with you. How do you go about reproducing that list? Introduce some meaningful grouping system. One method to use is grouping your list by category: What do you need in the way of fruits and vegetables, dairy products, laundry products, meats, and so on? If you go through all the categories in your mind, or imagine yourself walking down the aisles of the supermarket and passing the different organized sections of commodities, chances are you can do your shopping even without the list. Another sensible way to remember the missing shopping list is to organize it by purpose: Why are you going out shopping? Perhaps you have to shop for dinner for company. Then you can recreate your list by first course (get the pimentoes and anchovies for appetizer), second course (baking potatoes and sour cream to go with the steak), and third course (buy apple pie and ice cream, and don't forget some artificial sweetener for Joe).

When things are meaningful, you can remember them almost effortlessly; memory becomes difficult when material is meaningless or beyond your understanding. Take, for example, the following two lines. One is a sentence of nonsense words, the other is a sentence of meaningful words:

Lyk mij wuk bru gly por ilg der trum wappy lev efric blef hizdrl nugthrom zek.
Johnson owes me ninety-seven dollars and it's up to you to make him pay me back.

The nonsense words are impossible to remember, except with a great deal of effort. The meaningful words can be remembered immediately. What this means is that in order for you to remember something you must first understand it. Trying to remember material by rote, without making any sense out of it, takes enormous effort. Your time will be much more efficiently spent trying to make sense out of material than trying to remember it when it doesn't make sense. As soon as material becomes meaningful and intelligible it will find a place in your long-term memory.

Much of the material and information we want to remember is meaningful in and of itself, even though we may have trouble understanding it. A physics formula such as $V = d/t$ is meaningful, but if we do not understand what it means, it is as hard to remember as a nonsense syllable. When you are dealing with information of this sort, be it physics, math, history, appliance-operating instructions, or what have you, put your first effort into understanding the material. Only then does it make sense to try to store it in your memory bank. There is an expression in the computer field—GIGO—which means: *Garbage in, garbage out.* Applying this expression to your memory system, it means that if you try to store meaningless, unintelligible material in your memory system, you can only expect to end up with something worthless.

When other people seem to be able to remember seemingly meaningless information with ease, it is because they have been able to find a meaning in it which eludes you. Chess masters, for example, can glance at a board and remember the positions of all the pieces, or even the positions of all the pieces on five different boards at one time. This memory feat is made possible by their ability to organize the positions into patterns. The expert does not see individual pieces sitting on individual squares but sees total strategies in action, making memorization simple. To the nonplayer, the positions of the pieces are meaningless, hence not memorizable.

In the chapter "Processing Verbal Information," we discussed how to deal with new information to make it more meaningful. Here we only want to emphasize that you have to understand new information before you try to remember it. Once you have absorbed new material and have grasped its meaning, you then can focus on ways to file it away in your memory closet. To store it for easy retrieval, you want to put it in a sensible place with other similar memories so you can find it easily when you need it. First, always tell yourself, "I want to remember this," thereby consciously motivating yourself and directing your attention to the material to make it stick. Then ask yourself, "How do I want to file this information—under what headings?" The more you can connect a new piece of information to other pieces of information already tucked away, the better you will remember it. Suppose for example, you want to remember the information in this chapter. There are many ways to catalogue this material in your mind. Obviously, you can store the information under *memory* and what you already know about memory. You can also store some of the information under *seven* (things that come in groups of seven: seven things you can remember at once, seven days of the week, seven planets); or under *three* (important triads: the three divisions of the memory system, the three primary colors, the three divisions of matter in the universe); or under *attention* (attend to memories, attend and be alert, stand at attention, pay attention). And so on. It is also very important that you store the information away in its context—as part of the memory of you sitting in your chair and reading this book. When you are aware of your surroundings and situation as you are taking in new information, you will be able to remember that information better later by simply recalling the scene.

You probably have often had the experience of sitting quietly in a bus, room, office, or elsewhere and having your mind flooded with a series of thoughts and pictures. You do not have to work at this; the associations just flow. As you think of going to the movies last night, it reminds you of a different movie with Paul Newman and then you recall that when you saw the Newman movie you were with X and remember a discussion you had after the movie at Y's house about the meaning of risk in a person's life and the attraction of danger, which reminds you that you have to check the air in the tires, and so on. This typical sample of free association shows you how easily memories are stimulated when connected to other events. The lesson here is that the more you tie new information to other information you have already absorbed, the easier it will be to retrieve when you want it.

IMAGERY

So far we have mentioned three important aids to memory: attention, grouping, and organizing. There is a fourth that is just as important: imagery, or the ability to imagine something visually. Most people have very little trouble remembering visual material. You can probably conjure up in your mind right now the faces of your classmates in high school, or the waiting room at your dentist's office, but you probably would have a much harder time trying to remember the names of your classmates, or your dentist's phone number. Because visual material is so much easier for us to recall than verbal material, one of the best memory aids is to create a visual image of material you want to remember.

Take a shopping list again as an example. You can remember your shopping list better if you make it more vivid by visualizing the items on the list. Try to visualize the items listed on page 89 instead of just rehearsing them verbally. Picture in your mind your dinner table. See the service plate with potatoes covered with sour cream, and topped with anchovies and pimentos. Next to that is a dessert plate with ice-cream-topped pie, and the silver dish with artificial sweetener envelopes. When you literally can see what you have to buy, your list will stick in your mind.

Suppose you have been given driving directions to get to someone's house. You have written them down but you want to remember them because it will be dark when you are driving, making it difficult to read the instructions in the car. To remember the instructions, read them back to yourself, and visualize the route as you read it through. Picture yourself in the car, see yourself coming to the first stop light, now imagine you are putting on your turn indicator and making a left. Continue visualizing yourself driving the entire route—see yourself drive past the school, make a right turn one block later, look for the stop sign, and then the third house down the street. Once you rehearse the route visually, you will probably have no trouble at all remembering the instructions.

Visualization helps you remember more complicated material too. If you are reading a history text, for example, try to visualize the events described and create your own internal movie. If you're reading about World War I, imagine what Sarajevo must have looked like, try to picture Archduke Ferdinand, look for the assassin getting ready to shoot him, picture the aftermath, imagine people's reactions, and so on. If you're reading a book on animal behavior, try to picture the forest, the undergrowth, look for the animal burrows; try to visualize all the information that is being described verbally. Good texts include drawings, photos, maps, and diagrams, because visualization not only helps you to understand but also helps you to remember.

Imagery works best when you want to remember something concrete rather than conceptual, because it is easier to visualize a place, a person, or an object than it is to visualize an idea. You can still use visualization for remembering ideas and concepts, however, by trying to make the concepts concrete. For example, if you want to remember the various articles in the Bill of Rights—Article 1, religion, speech, press and assembly; Article 2, right to bear arms; etc.—translate these articles into visual situations. For Article 1 you might picture a minister giving a sermon in church, while some of the parishioners are reading the paper, emphasizing in your image that all are free to worship, speak, gather, and read what they want. For Article 2 you might visualize a train full of daily commuters all wearing holsters and pistols over their gray flannel suits, and so on. The sillier the image, the more it will stand out in your mind. It does not matter whether it is totally realistic, just as long as the image conveys the concept and makes a striking picture.

Not only are images a good memory aid in and of themselves, but they also work well in combination with other memory techniques. Always try to create a visual image for information you want to remember, and try to make that image vivid. It is more important that your image be distinctive and flashy than that it be completely accurate and realistic. Exaggerate, ham it up, and your image will work for you.

Images that you create should not be confused with so-called photographic memories. The former images are indirect, in that they are not sights you have actually seen, but rather pictures you concoct in your mind. Photographic memories are direct images of things actually seen. When you try to visualize your room, for example, it appears in your mind somewhat like a photograph, although it may be a badly lit photograph with the details rather hazy. Some people are able to see very distinct and accurate images—also referred to as *eidetic images,* from the Greek word for "that which is seen." Interestingly, children are much better eidetic imagers than adults and studies suggest that half of all children under eleven have eidetic images. It appears that this is a memory ability that is educated out of us as we mature and is usually lost by age fourteen. Other cultures, which rely less heavily on verbal education, have more eidetic imagers among adults and other adults show eidetic imagery when regressed under hypnosis, indicating that the power remains even though we may not know how to tap it.

Eidetic images differ from the usual direct images most of us experience in several ways. While we tend to see ordinary images of events or happenings in our minds, eidetic images are seen outside of the body, as if they were actually pictures in the space before us. Eidetic images are clearer than the usually experienced direct image, and, furthermore, they tend to hide the background against which they are seen as resting. These images last longer than normal images and have been recalled several months later. While looking at an eidetic image, the imager can see many accurate details that might not have been consciously noticed when originally viewing the scene. Imagers have also been able to move objects mentally in the image to see what they looked like from a different perspective.

MNEMONICS

Mnemonics, pronounced *ni-mon'iks*, comes from the Greek word for memory and means any technique that helps you remember better. Mnemonic devices were used in ancient Egyptian, Hindu, Greek and Roman civilizations and have come down to us from many sources. You probably know quite a few mnemonics yourself, like "*i* before *e* except after *c*," "thirty days hath September, . . ." and "Every Good Boy Deserves Food," which are, respectively, mnemonic devices for remembering spelling rules for i/e words, the number of days in each month, and the notes that appear on the lines of the music staff. Such techniques do not have a particularly good reputation, especially among teachers, who tend to think of mnemonics as akin to cheating. They feel that memory should be based on a solid understanding of the material and that mnemonics enable people to remember information without this understanding. Well, they are right and wrong. You need a solid understanding, but mnemonics are actually a way to introduce understanding where there is none. Memory devices provide a structure (and organization) for information that otherwise is too meaningless to be absorbed. The number of days in each month, for example, is quite arbitrary and therefore just as hard to remember as a list of nonsense syllables. The rhyme "Thirty days hath September, April, June, and November" brings some pattern into the arbitrary divisions and thereby enables people to remember the number of days in each month. All the mnemonic devices described here follow this same principle—they are designed to make meaningful patterns of meaningless information and to bring structure into chaos.

Rhymes and Rhythms

One of the most effective techniques for remembering information is to set it to rhyme. We already mentioned two such rhymes—"*i* before *e* except after *c*," and "thirty days hath September, April, June and November." Advertisers are well aware of the effectiveness of rhymes as memory devices and have bombarded us for years with jingle after jingle so that we remember to go out and buy their brands. When we were young, one of the first advertising jingles we heard was "You'll wonder where the yellow went when you brush your teeth with Pepsodent," and we still remember that as well as the parody jingle, "Pepsodent makes my teeth so clean my friends all think I'm using Gleem." Advertising jingles stick with us despite ourselves, but we can also put rhymes to use for our benefit. Whenever you have material to memorize that is difficult because it is not particularly meaningful or well structured, try to summarize it in a simple rhyme. To illustrate this we've put some of the information in this chapter into rhyme. If you want to remember the three stages of the memory process, try this:

Immediate memory, short-term and long
Are the stages that make a memory strong.

How about the phone number we mentioned before: 663–1514:

Six six three one five one four
I can't remember any more.

If you switch the number around to 663–1415 you can still make a rhyme:

Six six three one four one five
Can I remember all that jive?

How about reversing it to 151–4663?

One five one four six six three
This could be the death of me.

And so on. All sorts of unrelated pieces of information that you want to remember can be strung together in a rhyme of some sort that will help you to recall it when you want.

Acronyms

Acronyms have become a part of our daily life and are used so frequently because they are so effective. NATO, IBM, SST, and a host of other acronyms are not only economical ways of writing North Atlantic Treaty Organization, International Business Machines, and supersonic transport, but they also help us to remember what those longer names actually are. Acronyms have also been developed to help people remember lists of words or other pieces of data that do not meaningfully connect to each other; the acronyms provide a clue to the sequence and first letter of the material to be recalled. For example, to remember the notes that occupy the spaces of the music staff, one can try to keep in mind the letters, f, a, c, and e, or the acronym FACE. The notes that fall on the lines of the staff are harder to fit into an acronym—e, g, b, d, f—but they can be remembered in the acronym-like sentence we referred to before, "Every Good Boy Deserves Food."

The acronym method can be applied easily to any series that you want to remember. The colors in the spectrum for example, red, orange, yellow, green, blue, indigo, violet, can easily be recalled in their correct order if you translate them into an acronym like *Roy G Biv* or into the acronymic sentence used by English schoolchildren: "Richard Of York Gained Battles In Vain." Medical students, who have to remember the names of the olfactory, optic, oculomotor, trochlear, trigeminal, abducens, facial, auditory, glossopharyngeal, vagus, spinal accessory, and hypoglossal nerves, have for generations used the following acronymic-type rhyme:

On Old Olympus' Tiny Tops
A Finn And German Viewed Some Hops.

You can try making your own acronyms, using just the initial letter of each nerve name. Or suppose you want to remember the three stages of memory. You could make an acronym like LIST (long, immediate, short-term), SLIM (short, long, immediate memory), and so on. The important thing in making up an acronym is that it is simple and makes sense to you. You don't have to rely on ready-made acronyms to commit information to memory. Whenever there is a list of things you want to remember, make up your own acronym and you will find the list available to you whenever you want to call it up.

Exercise

Make up an acronym for the following items on a shopping list. You do not have to remember them in any special order: apples, eggs, ice cream, coffee, nuts, raisins, cheese, anchovies, lemons, limes. Some possibilities are: I CAN RECALL, CARL ELI CAN, CAN LIL RACE.

The Method of Loci

This method comes down to us from the Greeks. Loci, or locations, are used to remember things by assigning them a fixed position in space. You probably use a variant of this method already, although you may not be aware of it. For example, if we were to ask you how many windows there are in your house or apartment, you probably wouldn't remember, but if you take a mental walk through your home, going from room to room, you will very easily be able to see all the windows and count them. The method of loci can also be used for remembering other things, by associating them with particular places. First, decide on a predetermined sequence of locations. This could be a trip through your house (the cellar, the kitchen, the living room, the guest room, the staircase) or the places you pass on your way to work (the corner light, the newsstand, the little park, the funeral parlor, the bus stop, and so on). Once you have a route firmly in mind, use the different sites as mental places to put the items you want to remember. For example, suppose you want to remember a list of purchases to make at the supermarket: toilet paper, detergent, tuna fish, eggs, mayonnaise. Take each item and put it in a different spot on your walk to work. Then create vivid images of the items in their locations. Imagine the toilet paper wrapped around the traffic light, the detergent foaming out of the newsstand, cans of tuna fish lining the park walks, mayonnaise smeared over the caskets, sunnyside eggs plopped on the bus stop bench. When you get to the supermarket you merely have to imagine walking to work and the method of loci will do the rest.

The loci method enables you to remember because it lets you take a series of unrelated objects and recode them into a meaningful sequence of things—like the places you pass on the way to work or the rooms in your house. This method is used by all the memory experts to remember a vastly greater number of objects or ideas than would be possible if they tried to recall these things in and of themselves. You can also use the method to remember less mundane things than a shopping list. The Greeks, for example, used to remember major points in a speech by the method of loci, a habit which comes down to us in such expressions as "in the first place, and in the second place."

Peg Words

Peg-word systems are a variation of the method of loci. Instead of taking a mental walk through a familiar place where locations 1, 2, 3, and so on are designated by specific landmarks, you associate each of the numbers 1, 2, 3, etc. with a standard object or peg. Most memory experts use a set of objects that rhyme with the numbers they represent, as in the following list:

One is a bun.
Two is a shoe.
Three is a tree.
Four is a door.
Five is a hive.
Six is sticks.
Seven is heaven.
Eight is a gate.
Nine is a line.
Ten is a hen.

In using the peg-word system, the first step is to remember the associated number-object pairs until they become automatic. This is quite easy to do since the list incorporates the mnemonic device of rhyme. Just recite the rhymed pairs to yourself several times, and you will find them sticking in your mind.

Now for step two. Take the peg words and try out the same grocery list that we tried to remember with the method of loci: toilet paper, detergent, tuna fish, mayonnaise, eggs. The procedure is the same as before except this time, instead of associating the shopping list items with the places on our walk, associate them with the objects on the list: bun, shoe, tree, door, hive, etc. As you go from object to object, rather than place to place, it is important that you create the same type of vivid images used for the method of loci. Getting back to the list, toilet paper is the first item, and that goes with bun, so we could imagine a Mac· Donald's bun wrapped in toilet paper instead of the usual plastic box. Detergent is next and goes with shoe and we can have the bubbles coming out of the shoe this time. Tuna fish goes with the tree—perhaps you might want to visualize cans of tuna hanging from the tree. Mayonnaise is four—and it is spread all over the door. Eggs is five—maybe they are splattered on the hive. When you get to the supermarket, and repeat the rhyme to yourself— one is a bun, two is a shoe, etc.—you will see toilet paper, detergent, and the other objects before your eyes.

The method of loci and peg-word system have different kinds of applicability. The first is best when you want to remember relatively short lists of objects in order. The latter is good for lists if the order is not of prime importance or if you do not have to rattle off the list quickly.

Number-Consonant Equivalents

This method is probably the system most widely used by memory experts for remembering numbers. Words generally have more meaning to us than numbers, and this method provides a way to translate numbers into words. Each number is associated with a consonant that is similar in form to the number, as shown in the following chart:

Number	Similarly Shaped Consonant
1	t (1 downstroke)
2	n (2 downstrokes)
3	m (3 downstrokes)
4	r (last letter of 4)
5	l (Roman numeral for 50 is L)
6	j (mirror image of 6)
	or sh (sounds like j)
	or ch (sounds like j)

Number	Similarly Shaped Consonant
7	k (two 7s back to back)
	or q (sounds like k)
	or g (hard g sounds like k)
8	f (script f looks like 8)
	or v (similar in sound to f)
9	p (mirror image of 9)
	or b (reflection of p and similar in sound)
10 or 0	z (for zero)
	or s (similar in sound to z)

After you have memorized the number–consonant pairs, you are ready to apply the method. Instead of trying to remember them by rote, remember them in terms of their meaningful connection with each other. Once you have the pairs down pat, you can convert any number into a word, using the consonant equivalents and any vowels you need to flesh out a word. You can use any vowels to create your words, but the consonants must be the equivalents of your actual numbers.

An important phone number for you to remember is 911, the emergency number. Although it is simple, people tend to confuse it with the number for repairs (611) or for information (411). One way to help you keep it in mind is to translate it into a word: 911 is the same as the consonants P T T. By adding a few vowels in between those consonants we end up with PoTaTo, and if we think of a *hot potato* we think of trouble. Remembering the word *potato* is easy, and translating that back into 911 is also easy to do, once you have the system memorized. You just have to reconvert the consonants into numbers. You can remember how to distinguish 611 in the same way: 611 is the same as J T T; or SH T T; or CH T T. If we take the SH and put an i in between that and the two Ts, we get a word that you often feel like saying when your phone is out of order!

These two illustrations show how the method works, but often with such short numbers you do not need any mnemonic aids. This method comes in very handy for longer numbers, however. A few pages back we tried setting some phone numbers to rhyme for easier recall. Let's take those same numbers now and see how they can be remembered with the consonant method:

663–1514 equals SH SH M T L T R
663–1415 equals SH SH M T R T L

With the first group of consonants we could make up a phrase like SHoo SHoo My TooL TRee, and with the second we can alter that somewhat to read SHoo SHoo My TuRTLe. After you make up the words, create a clear image of them in your mind for extra effect and vividness. By this method we can keep both numbers in mind, and keep them from getting confused with each other.

Sometimes you have other numerical material to remember—heights of buildings for an engineering class, distances between cities for your work in a travel office, and so on. These bits of numerical information too can be effectively translated into words. Suppose you want to remember the heights of the Eiffel Tower, the Great Wall of China and the Empire State Building. The Eiffel Tower is 985 feet or B F L. That can convert to Boy FLy and gives you a vivid picture of a boy flying from the top of the tower. The Great Wall of China is thirty feet high or MZ. We can turn that into aMaZe and think of the people looking in amazement at the Great Wall. The Empire State Building is 1,250 feet high. We can translate that into eaT NaiLS, and imagine a strong, nail-eating King Kong sitting on top of the building.

Exercise

Here is a list of numbers that could represent anything at all—altitudes, distances, phone numbers. Your job is to translate these numbers into consonants and then into meaningful words and phrases that will be easy to visualize and remember.

10

646

248

1492

814–5260

243–2142

Some possibilities are: 10 = ToeS; 646 = CHuRCH; 248 = NeRVe; 1492 = TuRBaN; 814–5260 = aFTeR LuNCHeS; 243–2142 = No RooM No TRaiN.

Picture Equivalents

This method converts names, places, or ideas to be remembered into picture equivalents based on their sound or meaning. It is a particularly helpful system for remembering people's names and occupations. Let's see how it works.

A lot of people we know have trouble remembering the name Ehrenberg. To help recall it, you can use the picture equivalent method. First convert the name into similar sounding words that are familiar. You could, for example, convert Ehrenberg to Errand Bird, then visualize a bird delivering a package or message at the front door. Another possibility is to convert Ehrenberg to Erin Bird and you can visualize this as a bright green bird flying over Ireland. It does not so much matter what you convert a name to as long as you make a clear and distinctive picture from it. It will be much easier for you to remember the picture, and thereby recall the name, than to remember the name by itself.

After you try the technique with your name and the names of your friends, you will find it becomes easy to do, as well as fun. We have a friend whose last name is Nuetzel. For an exercise, see what you can think of right now to convert the name Nuetzel into a picture equivalent.

Some of the ones we have come up with are: Nude Sale, picturing a bunch of naked salespersons holding a flea market or, if you want, a sale of nudes; New Cell, a prison cell looking very new and tied up by a big red bow; Nut Shell, a giant walnut shell with our friend's face inside.

If you have trouble remembering people's names when you meet them, this method can be very helpful. When you are introduced, try quickly to form a picture equivalent, and then relate this image to something distinctive about the person's face.

To help you remember names, Harry Lorayne, a memory expert, has developed picture equivalents of 800 common American names. These are listed in *The Memory Book*, which he wrote in collaboration with Jerry Lucas. They suggest that you keep a file in your mind of people's titles and occupations—vice-president, general, accountant, etc.—so that you have picture equivalents handy to add on to the image of the name. Vice-president can be pictured as a vise, general as a star, accountant as a ledger, and so on.

This method is not restricted to names, even though it is very useful for that purpose. You can also apply it to learning foreign vocabulary. Suppose you want to learn the following Spanish words: *pato*–duck; *lápiz*–pencil; *caballo* (pronounced *cab-eye-o*)– horse; *mesa*–table. You could convert these pairs into picture equivalents by first finding an English word that sounds like the Spanish word. *Pato* (duck) sounds like pot, so we would picture a duck wearing a pot on its head. *Caballo* (horse) sounds like a cab going bye-o, so we could picture a horse waving its front hoof good bye-o to the cab. *Lápiz* (pencil) sounds like a lap, so we could picture someone's lap with a bunch of pencils in it.

Don't worry that your picture equivalents are not exact and a bit ludicrous. That just helps the memory process along.

Chains

The chain system is a good technique for remembering lists of objects or names in a particular sequence. Basically what you do is relate each item on the list to the item following it by means of associations that you create. This can be done in either one of two ways: the simple chain or the story.

Going back to the shopping list again, which you probably know by heart already, we had the following items: toilet paper, detergent, tuna fish, eggs, mayonnaise. To construct a chain we want to make vivid associations of each object to those connecting to it. Starting with toilet paper, we want to pair that with detergent. We could imagine rolls of unfurled toilet paper waving on a mast that is stuck in a billowing pile of detergent suds. Next we want to associate detergent with tuna fish. Perhaps we see tunas swimming in the detergent foam. Tuna fish must now be associated with eggs: each tuna is spitting out an egg from its mouth. For the egg-mayonnaise pair we could imagine eggs flying through the air, landing, and breaking into a dish and being whipped into mayonnaise.

Another way of linking these objects together is to create a story involving them all. Again, it can be wild and far out and that, in fact, will make it more memorable: Mary was at home writing her diary, which she kept on rolls of toilet paper because she felt all wound up. As she looked out the window she saw it was raining detergent flakes. Then the sun started to shine, creating a rainbow, which colored the flakes. As she looked closer she saw that the colored flakes were actually the scales on tuna floating in the air, so she knew something was fishy. She thought, "I better get a hold on myself. My vision is getting scrambled, so I'd better make some eggs and settle down." She went to the kitchen to fix her snack. "I'm spreading myself too thin," she told herself, "I'd better slap some mayonnaise on my bread and. . . ."

Because the chain system links the objects together, it is necessary to go through it link by link. This is fine when you want to remember lists in sequence, but the method is not particularly appropriate to other types of material.

THE IMPORTANCE OF TIMING

Our memory system works best when we are at a moderate state of arousal. On waking up in the morning we tend to be at a low level of arousal and not particularly alert to incoming sensory messages, making that a poor time to try to remember important material. Wait until you get going and perhaps have had a cup of coffee; if you can, give yourself a good hour to get properly alert before trying to memorize material. As the day passes, if you feel yourself drooping, don't place an extra burden on yourself by trying to work then at memorization. It is also a good idea not to work at remembering material when you are in a high state of arousal because it interferes with your ability to focus and transfer material to the short-term memory system. You can, of course, remember material you come across during any of these arousal states, but your task will be easier if you plan your time so that you can work at memory storage during moderate arousal times or at least leave the most difficult materials for these time periods.

Short-term memory deteriorates when you are tired, which tends to be at night; long-term memory is more efficient then, however, probably because long-term memory has a better opportunity to consolidate when we are in a low state of arousal and not processing too many incoming stimuli. What this suggests is that it is a good idea to process difficult new material through short-term memory during the early evening, and let the long-term memory consolidate as you get tired, go to sleep, and dream.

Just as general arousal of your nervous system is important to enhance your memory, specific arousal of your sensory register and information-processing channels also benefits your memory. It is a good idea to give yourself a warm-up period before you work at remembering new information—to grease the machinery, so to speak. You can exercise your memory processes by reviewing simple but similar material before you get down to serious work. If, for example, you want to work at memorizing a long poem, warm up by trying to remember first a few couplets. Or, if you want to memorize some difficult foreign phrases, warm up first by practicing some new, but fairly uncomplicated words. You can also warm up by reviewing similar material that you already know that relates to what you want to memorize. This not only helps the organizational process, but lets you start to work in the proper frame of mind.

Avoid working on memorizing new material for more than forty-five minutes at a time, even if this means interrupting yourself at a seemingly critical point. Your memory is actually enhanced when you are interrupted at these times. The tension created by such interruptions makes the material more memorable than material processed without a break. Five- to ten-minute breaks devoid of heavy mental activity will help to consolidate the long-term memory and give you the opportunity to enhance the primacy and recency effects.

Because new information takes time to consolidate and form a stable memory trace, it is a good idea, in order to prevent forgetting, to give yourself review periods after learning something new. The best timing for reviews is to coincide with the critical stages of the consolidation process. One consolidation period occurs at the time of transfer from short-term to long-term memory, when protein synthesis is occurring in the brain. Another point of consolidation seems to occur during sleep, particularly during dreams, when the day's material is reworked and more fully integrated. A third point of consolidation appears to occur a week or so after original learning, along with a permanent structural change in the brain. Arrange for a first review period five minutes after your exposure to the new material, a second review period a day later, and a third review period about a week later. Keep these reviews to five minutes each. If you are worried about the possibility of forgetting the new material, extra review periods at one month and six months later for two minutes each should serve to make it permanently available for retrieval.

WHY WE FORGET

A lot of what we attribute to memory loss is actually due to a lack of attention, meaning the information was never stored to begin with and simply isn't there to remember. If you try right now to draw a penny or a dollar bill and then match your drawing with the real thing, you will see how little you notice of the objects that you handle every day. We do not create memory traces when our minds are elsewhere and we are not paying attention. Memory problems primarily involve a difficulty of retrieval and can be helped by the methods of storage we discussed.

If our memory capacity is unlimited, why do we seem to forget? Several different factors are at work. One of the most prevalent problems is what is known as motivated forgetting, a concept that owes much to Sigmund Freud. Often, we appear to forget things when it is in our unconscious interest to do so. Unpleasant events and painful experiences that disturb our tranquility are frequently forgotten by our conscious minds. The victim or perpetrator of a violent crime will often be heard on the witness stand to say, "I can't remember what happened after that." This is not necessarily an alibi of the guilty party, since the offended party frequently suffers a similar memory loss. Such forgetting can be an unconscious attempt to protect the self from the necessity of reliving a difficult experience.

Similar to the total forgetting that can occur, people sometimes have partial and distorted memories that serve to soothe the ego. Thus, good times are remembered better than bad times, and pleasant aspects may be exaggerated in memory while unpleasant aspects are toned down. Memories can also be distorted when they are incomplete and we fill the gaps with details that seem reasonable to us and fit in with our biases.

Sometimes new information seems to interfere with our ability to remember old information. This phenomenon occurs when the new information is very similar to information already stored. Rather than actually crowding out the old information, what seems to happen is that the new information is not sufficiently differentiated from the old and the memories merge. Elizabeth Loftus, a psychologist at the University of Washington, has demonstrated experimentally that people alter old memories to accommodate new information. It also happens that new information seems to be quickly forgotten because of the interfering effects of succeeding events. In this case, consolidation of the new information in the memory bank is disrupted by the concurrent attempt at integrating the more recent stimuli. To avoid this type of forgetting you have to eliminate interfering events. For instance, it is a good idea to learn new material before you go to bed at night. Experiments have shown that people who go to sleep after learning material have better recall for the material than do people who carry on normal activities after the learning period. If it is not possible for you to sleep after taking in new information and you want to enhance your memory of it, take a rest break and do something mindless in that period. This gives the new information a chance to consolidate without interference.

People who go on alcohol binges often seem to forget a great deal. They report the morning after: "I can't remember a thing." Actually, their memories for past events are intact; they black out events dating from the time of their binge. What happens is that the alcohol interferes with the ability to store new memories and transfer them to long-term memory because the senses and cognitive processes are depressed. The only way that we know of overcoming this problem is to cut down on drinking. The most deleterious effects of alcohol come not from overall consumption of alcohol, but from concentrated consumption. One drink a day will not affect your memory, but seven drinks at one time will disrupt your memory processes and a lot more besides. We will say more about alcohol and its effects in the chapter on "The Care and Feeding of Your Brain."

Forgetfulness associated with old age and senility seems to come about as a problem in long-term memory storage. There is relatively little difference between young and old persons in short-term memory, but older people tend to have more difficulty retrieving material from long-term memory and organizing new material for storage. This appears to be a result of the physical process of aging and can be helped by proper care of the brain.

SUPER MEMORY

If you have ever studied a foreign language, you probably have no difficulty remembering how hard it was, but you probably *do* have difficulty remembering the foreign vocabulary and verb conjugations you learned. Now, keeping in mind how you struggled to learn Latin, French, Spanish, German, or whatever you studied, compare it to the effortless way you learned English. English came to you with no difficulty at all. The difference, apart from exposure time, stems primarily from the method of learning. When you were learning English your total mind was engaged and unencumbered by concerns about how well you were doing. You did not strain to learn, but absorbed the language in a relaxed, yet fully attentive, frame of mind. When you learned a foreign language, you were mentally less efficient, being impeded by worries about your ability to master it.

The super memory system tries to recreate the same kind of conditions that existed when you learned how to speak your native language and apply them to the learning and memorization of any new language or other material. This method, called Suggestopedia by its developer, Dr. Georgi Lozanov of Bulgaria, combines several techniques to induce a frame of mind that facilitates a greater absorption of information. Through positive suggestion, it releases you from the self-limiting attitudes you have been conditioned to accept about your learning abilities. It induces a relaxed state that frees your mind for total availability; it presents material to be learned in a tempo that is synchronized with your mind and body rhythms; it provides a background of music that induces an altered state of consciousness to increase your receptivity to the material to be remembered.

The super memory method is very popular in Eastern Europe and has been used in selected schools in the United States. Typical claims are that it speeds up learning five to ten times and that foreign languages are acquired in about one month. The method is suitable for memorizing factual material of any nature, but particularly helpful for material that is hard to remember such as foreign words, anatomy terms, biology classifications, numerical data, names and addresses of business contacts, and so on. If you would like to read more about this method and its rationale, look at *Superlearning* by Sheila Ostrander and Lynn Schroeder.

You can follow the super memory system on your own. All you need are two tape recorders, a written copy of the material you want to remember, and two recorded tapes that you will have to prepare yourself—one of music and one of the material you want to remember. If you want to remember more material, you will need more learning tapes.

Prepare your music tape on a ½-hour cassette from prerecorded records or tapes of Baroque music by a composer such as Bach, Corelli, Telemann or Vivaldi. Selections must be written in 4/4 time and recorded at a tempo of about sixty beats to the minute. Many largo sections of concerti are recorded at this speed, but check out the timing with a clock or metronome. Also check the adagio and larghetto movements. You will need to record a minimum of six or seven selections of appropriate music to give you about twenty minutes of music.

Record the material you want to remember on a separate tape. The material must be recited onto the tape rhythmically, in eight-second (8-beat) cycles of four seconds silence, four seconds information. This will correspond to the tempo of the music you have recorded. You don't have to read in time to the beats, but you have to record within the four seconds. Work with a clock to pace your recitation so you can fit the information into the four seconds. Try to vary your tone as you record, alternating from soft to normal to loud. Record about fifteen to twenty minutes' worth of material.

Super memory sessions should be preceded by review of the material you want to remember. The next preparatory step is relaxation exercises such as those described in the chapter "Emotions and Intelligence." When you are relaxed, recite self-affirming statements to yourself such as "I can do it"; "Remembering is easy for me." Continue to warm up for your super memory session by breathing rhythmically to slow your body and mind to calmer and more efficient levels. Your breathing rate should be synchronized with the pace of the learning materials: inhale and hold breath for four seconds while material is read on tape, exhale for a count of two during silence, inhale for the remaining two counts, then hold breath again for four counts while material is being read.

The super memory session itself is conducted in two parts. First listen to the memory tape and read over the material at the same time, breathing in time to the tape. As soon as the tape is finished, dim the lights, put on the music tape and replay the memory tape at the same time. Play the music at low volume to sustain a restful state. Sit back with your eyes closed, paying attention to what is being said, and breathing in time to the delivery. Try visualizing the material as you hear it, but be careful not to strain. As with any newly learned material, it will be helpful for memory storage if you review the material at the intervals suggested in the section on "Importance of Timing."

MODES OF THINKING

We use the word *thinking* to mean lots of different things: a flow of associations ("A penny for your thoughts"); an opinion ("What do you think about that?"); a doubt as opposed to a certainty ("I *thought* I saw her"); or a review of events ("I was just thinking about dinner last night"). In these thinking activities, thoughts just seem to come to us; ideas, remembered events, facts flow through our minds in what has been called a stream of consciousness. Thinking also means concentrated effort applied to problem-solving ("Sh, I'm busy thinking"; "He's deep in thought"). This chapter concentrates on deliberate thinking, which doesn't just come to you but which you make happen. This kind of thinking, which involves grasping ideas, understanding patterns, and applying rules of operation, makes it possible for you to elaborate on the information you already have on hand and thereby to generate new solutions.

CONCEPTUAL THINKING

Concepts are a basic tool of thinking and your adeptness in concept formation influences how well you can think. A concept represents the similarities in otherwise diverse objects, situations, or events. By bringing together in a single idea what we have learned about many different things, concepts enable us to think more effectively.

As children our initial concepts revolve around objects. We learn, for example, that caramels, chocolate bars, and gumdrops share enough attributes to form one concept, labeled *candy,* and that candy, cake, and ice cream share enough attributes to form the higher order concept of *dessert.* Having this concept, we can respond to a multitude of disparate-looking objects in the same way, namely by yearning for them and eating them. As we get older we also learn concepts that relate to feelings and situations, such as love, anger, play, bedtime, separation. Each of these concepts is a form of shorthand that condenses our past experiences into a single idea that helps us think more efficiently. Some shorthand systems are, however, better than others.

One common way of classifying objects or experiences is in terms of their particular meaning to the people involved. A person might, for example, classify a knife, spoon, plate, butter, loaf of bread, salt and pepper, and a flower vase together because he had all those things on the breakfast table. Since this classification does not relate directly to the characteristics of the objects, but to the situation of the individual, it is not a very useful thinking tool, having little validity when removed from the personal situation. A more intelligent concept is one that relates to the intrinsic qualities of the objects. Accordingly, we could classify the objects as eating utensils (knife, spoon, plate); food (butter, loaf of bread); condiments (salt and pepper); and decorative objects (flower vase). These classifications are universally understandable and serve as more meaningful bases for thinking.

Concepts that relate to the concrete qualities of objects are usually less useful than concepts that relate to their abstract qualities. To say that a tangerine and carrot belong together because they share the same concrete characteristic of orangeness is not as meaningful as to say that they share the same abstract quality of nutritiousness. The higher the level of abstraction of a concept, the more it captures the essence of elements within it. Plato said, "The lowest form of thinking is the base recognition of the object. The highest, the comprehensive intuition of the man who sees all things as part of a system."

Exercise

For each pair of words listed below, write down the way in which they are similar to each other. Search for their abstract qualities and higher-order similarities.

Items	How are they similar?
1. truck–car	
2. clock–scale	
3. butter–scrambled eggs	
4. beginning–end	
5. sad–happy	
6. flea–redwood	
7. garbage collector–governor	
8. dictatorship–democracy	

Now let's analyze some answers.

1. *Truck–car:* One common answer for the first pair is that truck and car are similar because they both have wheels (concrete characteristic). Another is that they are both means of transportation (abstract characteristic). Both answers are correct but the abstract answer is more intelligent. It enables us to enlarge the group and still have a sensible collection of objects. If we wanted to enlarge the group on the basis of wheels we could include truck, car, spinning wheel, water wheel, roulette wheel. These objects, while all having wheels, do not make a useful group. If we extend the group in terms of the concept "means of transportation," we could have truck, car, plane, boat and cable car. These objects do not all share wheels, but they share something more essential; that is, we can use them to get from one place to another.

2. *Clock–scale:* One answer is that they belong together because they both have pointers and faces with numbers. Another answer is that they belong together because they are measuring instruments. The better answer is, again, the one based on abstraction of their essential function.

3. *Butter–scrambled eggs:* The usual answers are that these items are similar because they are both yellow, because they are both eaten at breakfast, because the eggs are cooked in butter, because they both contain cholesterol, or because they are both dairy foods. Which is the best answer? The fact that they are both yellow, while correct, is not a meaningful concept, being limited to a concrete, superficial characteristic. That they are both eaten at breakfast is a situational concept that does not apply to all people and certainly not to people in different cultures. The answer that eggs are cooked in butter does not pinpoint any similarity or shared characteristic of those two items but merely states how one may act on the other. The answer "they both contain cholesterol" recognizes an essential similarity, and the answer "they are both dairy foods" is an even more useful concept because it includes the concept of cholesterol as well as the most essential common factor—that they are both food.

4. *Beginning–end:* People often have difficulty seeing any similarity between these two words, regarding them as opposites. Nevertheless, they do share the quality of being extreme positions, defining the outside limits.

5. *Sad–happy:* This is another pair that frequently gives difficulty because they seem to be opposites rather than concepts
that have anything in common. Although the feelings signi-
fied by these two words are opposites, they are both feelings
or emotional states.

6. *Flea–redwood:* One frequent response to this pair is that they
are similar because they are both found outdoors. This is
correct, but does not get at an essential similarity between a
flea and a redwood tree. For instance, flag poles, basketball
hoops, garbage cans, and traffic lights are also found outdoors, yet these objects do not seem to have much in common
with a flea and a redwood. A more intelligent response is that
a flea and redwood are both living things, since this relates to
their inherent characteristics rather than to their location.

7. *Garbage collector–governor:* Some people say these two terms
are similar because they both start with a *g*. This is, of course,
true but is a very limiting response, having little to do with
the basic nature of either term. It confuses the label with the
objects named. Another response is that a governor and a
garbage collector are both men. This may once have been the
case, but is no longer so. Even so, the terms *governor* and
garbage collector do not describe categories of people as much
as they describe occupations of people. A more apt response is
that these terms are similar because they both represent civil
service employees.

8. *Dictatorship–democracy:* The fact that these words both begin
with *d* is irrelevant, as we saw above, because that is a similarity in the labels, not in the things labeled. Although there
is a tendency to see these two words as representing things
that are different rather than things that share something in
common, both are the same in that they represent forms of
government.

Many intelligence tests contain a section on similarities or
concept identification and rate your responses according to the
criteria we discussed. The more abstract your concepts, the better
your score will be.

While the more abstract concepts generally lead to more
intelligent thinking, it is also important that you are able to
form concepts along a variety of dimensions and to switch
among them depending on the requirements of the situation.
Sometimes one quality of an object or experience is relevant, and

sometimes a different quality can be of greater relevance. If you arrive at a gathering at the community center and are looking for a date, it makes sense to classify the people on the basis of sex and to spend your time with one group or another, as the case may be. If you are there to run for elective office, you might want to classify people in terms of their political attitudes. If you were a visitor from outer space, you would want to classify all the people together as distinct from the inanimate objects so you would know from where you could obtain information about earth. Flexibility in conceptualization allows you to think more appropriately.

Exercise

Here is a list of objects. Take paper and pencil and write down separate lists of all the objects you think belong together, using as many different concepts for combining them as you can. You can put an object in more than one group.

wristwatch	lined paper
man	matches
zebra	striped shirt
smoking furnace	ruler
haystack	lit pipe
apple	cow

Let's take a look at some of the classifications that can be made:

wristwatch–ruler (measuring instruments)
smoking furnace–lit pipe (having fire)
lined paper–striped shirt–zebra (having stripes)
zebra–cow (animals, quadrupeds, mammals)
zebra–cow–man (animals, mammals, living creatures)
matches–ruler–pipe (made of wood)
matches–ruler–striped shirt–pipe (made of plant pulp or fibers)
haystack–apple (animal food, plant category)
wristwatch, smoking furnace, lined paper, striped shirt, ruler, lit pipe (manufactured objects)

When we think, we usually are called upon to use more than one concept at a time. To illustrate that point, let's consider card-playing. A deck of cards varies on three dimensions: suit, color, and value. If you are playing Go Fish, only one dimension is important, namely, value: one needs four threes, or four tens, or four of any particular value. Most other card games require that you employ at least two concepts at once. In bridge and poker both value and suit are essential. In solitaire, value, color, and suit are essential. Most of your thinking requires the integration of many different concepts. If you are wondering whether to pick up your daughter after school or let her come home by herself, you don't base a decision solely on your concept of parental role. Also essential to your decision are your concepts of self-reliance, maturational level, safety, and so on. In any thinking activity, whether playful or not, the ability to integrate two or more concepts into one is essential to intelligent thinking.

Though many concepts are handed down to us, we are constantly modifying our concepts to incorporate new experiences. We use new concepts to understand people (hardhats, hippies); personality types (laid back, uptight); music (acid rock, disco); films (cinéma verité, new wave); technological developments (gene-splicing, computer programming); international relations (terrorism, overkill); and every other aspect of life. Ready-made concepts are essential to our understanding of the world, but we also have to keep open to the possibility of discerning relationships on our own and forming new concepts. Creative ideas stem from the ability to develop such new concepts, discovering relationships among things that have not been discerned before.

MAKING HYPOTHESES

When faced with a problem, you can go about solving it in a hit-or-miss fashion, randomly trying one approach after another, or you can try to solve the problem by making hypotheses about what is likely to work and what is not. By using the latter method, you can reason out a solution based on the available information, saving time and effort. Suppose you are riding along a highway on your way to visit Washington, D.C. Because of a recent accident, the road sign is down and when you come to a three-way division of the road, you don't know which way to turn. One way to go about it is to take pot luck and pick a road at random. If this choice proves wrong, you can always come back and try two more times but the trial-and-error approach is not very economical either of your time or your gas, not to speak of your patience. A better method is to try to reason out the possibilities. To do this, collect all the available information so that you can make a choice that has a better probability of being correct. What is the available information in this instance? The pattern of traffic on these three roads. You can make reasonable inferences about where the three roads lead by observing which cars go where. Suppose the trucks mostly go to the middle road and the passenger cars and buses move to the right or left. You know that Washington, D.C., is not a dense residential district and contains no industry; therefore, you can safely assume the trucks are bypassing the city.

Hypothesis 1: The middle road is a city bypass. To continue with possibilities, people in the passenger cars are probably either on their way home or are tourists going to Washington, D.C., like you. You observe again. The cars with local plates, from Virginia or Maryland, are mainly going off on the road to the right. This probably means that these are residents on their way home.

Hypothesis 2: The road to the right leads to the city environs. To continue with this reasoning, if the out-of-state cars, like yours, and the buses, are going to the left, chances are that is the route to the capital.

Hypothesis 3: The left road leads to Washington, D.C. You might still be wrong, but at least now there is a better chance of being correct than there was before, and a reasonable basis on which to make your choice.

After you make your hypotheses, your next job is to test them to see which are right. Various strategies can be employed, some more effective than others. There are both direct and indirect tests as well as tests that allow you to test one, as opposed to more, hypotheses at a time.

Let's take a very simple example. Suppose you are on a job interview and the receptionist tells you to walk down the corridor and enter the personnel director's door at the end of the hall. When you get there, you find that there are two doors, not one. Peering inside, you notice one office is rather messy with lots of papers strewn about, while the other is very neat and tidy. Your hypothesis is that the neat office is the personnel director's. The direct test of your hypotheses would be to enter that office and ask, "Are you the personnel director?," but this might make a bad impression. The personnel director might think you forgot or misunderstood the directions, rather than thinking that the receptionist gave you sloppy instructions. Here it might be better to make an indirect test of your hypothesis by going to the door you assume is the wrong office and asking there, "Are you the personnel director?" If, as you assume, this is the wrong office, the occupant will send you next door and you can meet the personnel director without any loss of face. Let's take another example and see how direct and indirect tests work.

Exercise

You are shopping in a clothing store and notice a big counter sale on sweaters. The sign says, "Wool and Acrylic Sweaters, Some Imperfects." If you can find some first-quality wools, they are a very good buy, and you would like to purchase a whole bunch of them for Christmas presents, but you don't want any acrylics or imperfect wools. Judging by the low price, your hypothesis is that the wool sweaters must be imperfect. All the sweaters are neatly folded and wrapped in plastic bags, and each one has a tag inside the wrapping, with either the *contents* side facing up (wool, or acrylic), or the *quality* side facing up (seconds, first quality). You know the clerk will not let you unwrap more than two sweaters to check the underside of the tags, so which two tags will you turn over to test your hypothesis that the sweaters marked *Wool* are also marked imperfect? Many turn over two wool tags to see what is on the reverse. This is a direct test of the hypothesis, but even if it confirms your hunch, it is not too helpful because those two sweaters are not enough to establish the rule. Another solution, also a direct test, is to turn over one tag marked *Wool* and one marked *Imperfect*. This is a slightly better approach and, if both answers are in line with your hypothesis, you are apt to feel surer that you are correct in your hunch. The best test, though, is a combination of the direct and indirect approaches: you can turn over a tag marked *Wool* and one marked *Perfect*. If the wool tag reads *Imperfect* on the other side, and the *Perfect* tag reads *Acrylic* on the other side, you are on much firmer ground. Your hypothesis has two sides to it: that all wool sweaters are marked *Imperfect*, and that only acrylic sweaters are marked *Perfect*. If you can at the same time demonstrate both of these statements to be true, the probabilities are with you.

So far we have given examples of the importance of making hypotheses, and two different ways of testing them: the direct and the indirect. It is also a good idea to keep yourself flexible and to be ready to make up more than one hypothesis so that you can test different reasonable hypotheses at the same time.

Exercise

Below is a list of number groups. Each set of numbers is based on the same principle. Your job is to determine what principle was used. Look at the first five sets:

2–4–6
14–16–18
6–8–10
20–22–24
26–28–30

What is the principle? You probably decided that the rule is: starting with any even number, add 2 each time. That is one relation between the numbers, but not the one we had in mind. Look at the sixth and seventh sets and see if you can figure out the rule:

9–11–13
1–3–5

You might think that, starting with any number, odd or even, the principle is to add 2 each time. This is true of the numbers given, but not the principle being used, as you can see by the number sets below:

8–12–16
5–20–35
0–7–14
1–50–99

It's obvious now that the difference between the numbers can vary. Maybe the rule is that whatever the difference between the first two numbers is, the same difference holds between the second and third numbers. That describes the numbers given, but is not the rule. Perhaps then, the rule is that the middle number is always the average of the other two? That also describes the number series given, but is still not the correct rule. Look at the next examples and see if you can figure out the rule that applies to them as well as to all the number series given so far:

3–7–12
25–27–30
1–4–10

The answer is simple. The rule is any three numbers in order of magnitude. This is not a trick, but an easy problem to solve if you made several hypotheses about it rather than just one. Usually, when people arrive at one hypothesis that makes sense, they stop thinking and do not bother to test other possibilities. That way, easy solutions can be bypassed, while you go off pursuing more complicated hypotheses.

VISUAL THINKING

Thinking is often aided by the ability to visualize the problem. Because problem solutions so often come to us through visual images, we use such expressions as "I see what you mean," and "I get the picture," to indicate understanding. The importance of this principle has been recognized in education by the use of visual aids to help you understand the problem. Remember back to your geometry class for a minute. Can you imagine how difficult it would have been if you hadn't drawn diagrams of all those triangles and circles and tried to work out solutions only from a verbally stated problem? Look at the following two ways of stating a geometry problem. The problem in word form is a complicated mess:

If you have a straight line with points ACDB on it, in that order, and AD = CB, prove that AC = DB.

Once put into visual terms, the problem is easy to understand and solve:

AD = CB Prove AC = DB

$$\overline{\underset{A \quad\quad C \;\; D \quad\;\; B}{\cdot \quad\quad\; \cdot \;\; \cdot \quad\;\; \cdot}}$$

When you see the problem in front of you, it is·clear that AD is the same as AC + CD, and that CB is the same as CD + DB. Since you know AD = CB, then AC + CD = CD + DB, and AC must equal DB (once you subtract CD from both sides of the equation).

Whenever you are faced with a problem, first try to visualize it before working on a solution. Sometimes this may mean drawing a picture, sometimes making a line with points on it, sometimes making a chart, and sometimes conjuring up an image before your eyes. One method of visualizing is to try to see yourself in the problem situation, as if you were actually a part of it. The most famous example of this type of visualization is that of Einstein, who was aided in the development of the theory of relativity when he pictured himself riding on a beam of light with a mirror before him. Once he visualized himself on the beam, he realized he could not see his image because he and the mirror were moving at the speed of light, making it impossible for his image to reach the mirror. We know people who have tried to figure out how a series of gears will move by picturing themselves as one of the gears turning, and others who have tried to learn how to park a car by seeing themselves as the actual car being steered. Try a few exercises using different visualization methods.

Exercise

Problems involving directional orientation are particularly amenable to visualization. They are both easy to map out and simple to solve when visualized. Suppose you are touring a city and ask the hotel clerk for directions to the museum, which run as follows: "When you leave the hotel go left over the bridge, go straight for two blocks, then turn right, walk three more blocks and then turn left for two more blocks and the entrance is at the corner." If you draw yourself a map you can easily see how to get to the museum.

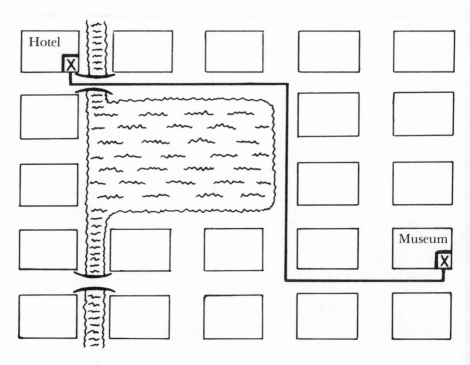

People who are adept at visualizing often do not need to draw a map but can see the form of the route they should follow. In this case it would be a Z route:

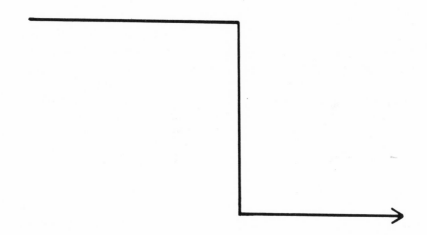

Exercise

There is a famous problem, designed by psychologist Karl Duncker, which goes basically like this: A person is suffering from an inoperable tumor which can, however, be treated with X ray. The trouble is that the strength of the X ray needed to kill the tumor will also kill the surrounding tissue, and put the person at risk. How do you treat this person? When Duncker presented this problem, he had people think it out. We have sketched the problem so you can visualize it and perhaps thereby also see the solution:

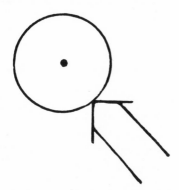

The tumor is encased by the body, and the strong ray can destroy the tissue it passes through as well as the tumor.

While studying the problem, try solving it not by thinking about it, but by trying to draw it differently. What can you change in the drawing? You cannot change the person, or the tumor, so that leaves the X ray. How can you change the way we drew the X ray? Approaching the problem this way lets you visualize the solution. Instead of drawing one thick line, you can draw many slender lines which, added together, will equal the same quantity, like so:

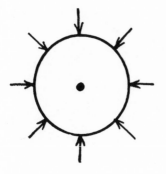

The tumor is bombarded by many weak X rays, which converge at the point of the tumor. None is strong enough to damage the surrounding tissue, but their combined strength is powerful enough to destroy the tumor.

Another possible solution involves the person. Although you cannot alter the person, if you look at the drawing it becomes apparent that you can alter the person's position relative to the X ray. This has the same effect as using many weak X rays that combine to focus on only one point where they can destroy the tumor.

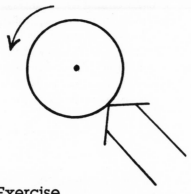

As the person rotates, the strength of the X ray on the outer tissue is momentary, but it remains concentrated at the center.

Exercise

Using the same approach, try to draw your way out of this problem, which was developed by Edward de Bono, about whom we will talk more later on. According to the laws of physics, all bodies fall at the same rate of speed. Suppose you had a small metal ball and a large one five times its size like those drawn below. Just by redrawing the problem, how can you demonstrate that they must fall at the same rate?

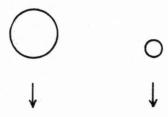

What can you change in this drawing? The only thing you have are two metal balls, so obviously one of them has to change. You can't make the small one bigger—that would be changing the problem by changing the mass, but you can make the big one smaller: visualize the big one as being equal to five small ones. Let's redraw it that way:

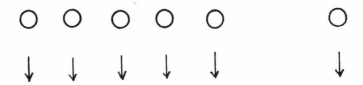

Now you can see that both objects fall at the same rate of speed, since they are basically the same—one is just a conglomeration of the other.

The importance of visualizing will become more apparent later, when we discuss creative thinking. Practically every person who has come up with an important new idea has reported visualizing the idea rather than thinking it out verbally. Keep trying this approach on all problems you have to work out. We have given you examples for visualizing that are drawn and can be presented on the pages of a book, but there are other ways of visualizing problems so that you can see them. Making 3-D models, as architects and engineers do; drawing plans to scale; making charts, maps, graphs, or hierarchies—all those are helpful visualizing tools. Which one you want to use will depend, of course, on the problem and how important the solution is to you.

ANALOGIES

An analogy is a comparison between two things. Sometimes problems and their solutions become simplified if you can make an analogy between the problem that is troubling you and another situation that you are familiar with and that has already been solved. When Leonardo da Vinci and the Wright Brothers wanted to fly, they looked at the birds and designed flying machines with wings. When Alexander Graham Bell developed the telephone, he followed the mechanism of the ear. Almost all inventions, from the great to the simple, have been based on analogy.

Analogies also can help in the understanding of concepts. The process of evolution, for example, can be grasped easily through the analogy of a tree branching out into different species. The process of incubation has jocularly been conveyed through the analogy of a cake in the oven. Psychoanalysis has been explained by likening it to peeling an onion: you keep penetrating deeper to the core of the personality, peeling off one layer after another. A psychotic outburst is often explained by analogy with a pressure cooker: if there is too much steam (tension) bottled up inside, the top (emotional control) will blow.

Analogical thinking does not have to be limited to the real, but can incorporate the fantastic as well. The idea of a people-mover or belt such as is used at many air terminals is easily conceptualized from the idea of the magical flying carpet. Look for the ideal solution to the problem, even if it means suspending what you know of the laws of nature, and search your fantasies for analogies. The creators of science fiction, in their wildest fantasies provided the idea for much of the space technology that is now taken for granted.

Try to use analogical thinking when facing a problem by making a comparison with something you know. The best analogies are usually those drawn from nature. Your own body and the way it works can provide the basis for analogies to many problems.

Exercise

Design an efficient mail delivery system for your town or postal district. Would it have a central mail office, mail offices at various road junctions, mail delivered by people on foot, in cars, by pneumatic tubes? How would outgoing mail be handled? As currently done, by pickups coordinated with mail deliveries, or some other way? What delivery system in nature can give you some clues for your design? How about basing the mail delivery and pickup system on the same design as your circulatory system?

LOGICAL REASONING

Logical reasoning is the process of making inferences about one set of statements or facts based on another set of statements or facts. For example, if you know that the temperature around the equator is hot, and that the Philippines lie on the equator, you do not have to go to the Philippines to find out what the weather is like. You can conclude through logic that the Philippines are hot. Although logic is very useful in increasing intelligence by allowing us to draw conclusions from certain premises, without the necessity for direct experience, it can also get in the way of greater intelligence. Behind this paradox lies the fact that logic is only a method for analyzing the relationship between statements and does not take into consideration the truth or meaningfulness of those statements. You can be logical and wrong at the same time.

Probably you are familiar with the following syllogism:

All men are mortal.
Socrates is a man.
Therefore Socrates is mortal.

In this instance, we not only grasp the validity of the conclusion and how it follows logically from the first two statements, but the statements themselves are obviously true. Using this same form, however, we can put together a different syllogism:

Whatever helps the economy is good for the citizenry.
Cigarette smoking helps the economy.
Therefore cigarette smoking is good for the citizenry.

In this second syllogism, although the conclusion is logically valid, it is false. If we reason from faulty premises, like the first one, we can end up with faulty but logical conclusions. Being logical is no guarantee of being right. Seeing the pitfalls of logic can help keep you from faulty reasoning and from being taken in by other people's faulty reasoning. Logic is irrelevant if you start from questionable premises.

A related problem is that the truth of statements can sometimes obscure that they do not follow logically from each other. Look at the next group of statements:

The nicotine and tars in cigarettes are bad for your health.
Chewing tobacco contains nicotine and tars.
Therefore chewing tobacco is bad for your health.

If we tend to agree with each statement we are likely to ignore the fact that the conclusion is invalid. The first premise only tells us about the harmfulness of tars and nicotine in cigarettes, not about the harmfulness of tars and nicotine in general, and so the conclusion does not logically follow although it is very reasonable. Again, logic and truth do not necessarily coincide.

Some forms of logical inference are much more difficult to follow than others. Two British psychologists, P. C. Wason and P. N. Johnson-Laird, among others, have conducted series of experiments to see how people work with different forms of logical inference; they have determined which forms give us the most trouble. Many people make errors when dealing with conditional inferences—a sequence of statements in the form "If . . . then," as in the following:

> If it sleets (A), then the roads will be icy (B).
> It is sleeting (A).
> Therefore, the roads are icy (B).

Conditional inferences have two parts: the *antecedent* or *if* part (A), and the *consequent* or *then* part (B). The simple form above is known as *affirming the antecedent,* which means that the second statement confirms that the *if* part is so. A related pattern of inference, known as *denying the consequent* is harder for most people to follow:

> If it is sleeting (A), then the roads will be icy (B).
> The roads are not icy (not B).
> Therefore, it is not sleeting (not A).

In this sequence, the second statement denies that the consequence has occurred. People have difficulty appreciating that this is a valid argument; the presence of the negative, as we discussed in the chapter "Processing Verbal Information," interferes with our ability to handle information.

Greater difficulty sets in when people have to deal with two other variations of the conditional argument. The first is known as *affirming the consequent,* in which the second statement confirms that the consequence has occurred.

> If it is sleeting (A), then the roads will be icy (B).
> The roads are icy (B).
> Therefore, it is sleeting (A).

Although the conclusion sounds reasonable, it is not logical. The first statement does not imply that the streets are icy only if it is sleeting. The streets could be icy if it had rained and the temperature suddenly dropped, or if it had snowed. The statement only lets us draw conclusions about what happens if it is sleeting, not about what accounts for icy roads. Thus, affirming the consequent is a logical fallacy.

The other fallacy, known as *denying the antecedent* (where the second statement denies that the *if* is so) is as follows:

If it is sleeting, then the roads will be icy (B).
It is not sleeting (not A).
Therefore, the roads are not icy (not B).

Here again, the first statement does not imply that only sleet can cause icy streets; the conclusion is therefore invalid.

In addition to problems with conditional inferences, many of us have difficulty with quantified inferences or those involving the quantity of things, such as *all, most, many, some* or *none*. Look at the following syllogism, for example:

	Basic Form
Some professors (A) are musicians (B).	Some A are B
No inventors (C) are professors (A).	No C are A
Therefore some musicians (B) are not inventors (C).	Some B are not C

People tend to think that this conclusion is not valid, although it is. The difficulty with quantified syllogisms is greatly reduced if they deal with familiar material. Thus, if we use the same form of syllogism as the above but write it in terms of familiar facts, the logic becomes apparent:

	Basic Form
Some mammals (bats) can fly.	Some A are B
No birds are mammals.	No C are A
Therefore some flying animals are not birds.	Some B are not C

When you have to reason through problems in the form of quantified syllogisms, first try to translate the argument into terms that are familiar to you. You may feel it is unlikely that you will run across problems of this type in the usual course of affairs, but quantified inferences tend to pop up in discussions all the time. For example, when the Equal Rights Amendment was being debated, we heard arguments like the following:

Some housewives do not want to work.
All working women will be financially insecure under ERA.
Therefore no housewives will be financially secure under ERA.

There are hundreds of different ways quantified statements can be arranged, but only a handful are logically valid. You can, of course, always check out a logic textbook to see what is logical and what is not logical, or you can try to figure it out yourself. The easiest way to reason through problems of quantified syllogisms is to translate the argument into terms that are familiar to you. Then the logic or illogic of the statements can be more easily realized.

Exercise

Determine whether the following syllogisms are valid or invalid. Try substituting statements you know are true for the As, Bs, and Cs. You can use the bats and mammals if you like, or any other categories that you feel comfortable with, like "All alcohol is intoxicating," "Some drinks are alcoholic," and so on.

1. Some A are B.
   All B are C.
   Therefore no A are C.
2. No A are B.
   Some B are C.
   Therefore some C are not A.
3. All B are A.
   Some B are C.
   Therefore some A are C.

The first conclusion is invalid, the second is valid, and the third is valid.

Sometimes it is easier to deal with quantified syllogisms if you try to visualize them, as in the circle diagrams developed by the Swiss mathematician, Leonhard Euler. A circle is used to represent different objects, with separate and detached circles indicating no members in common, overlapping circles indicating some members in common, and an enclosed circle indicating all members of the enclosed circle are a class included in the outer circle:

No A are B.

Some A are B.

All A are B.

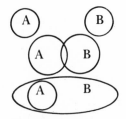

NATURAL REASONING

To think intelligently, we need to reason realistically as well as logically. Logical reasoning, as we saw, can be correct but lead to erroneous conclusions because it disregards the truth of its statements. It tells us whether or not one statement derives from another but not if that statement is plausible or if it is at all important. According to the rules of logic we can deduce that if an apple is red, it is also true that an apple is not green, but while the first fact tells us something important, the second is not very useful and is not a natural way to think.

Natural reasoning is not bound by any particular method but uses many approaches to help us evaluate ideas and determine their plausibility. This type of reasoning not only lets us make inferences from what we already know, but allows us to produce new knowledge by reordering our past experiences into new patterns. Instead of focusing on the rules for handling information, we focus on information itself. This lets us see more, play with hunches, and explore possibilities.

Imagine the situation of a teacher who is faced with a boy in her class who does not seem to be able to learn anything. She wants to know what is behind the problem so it can be dealt with appropriately. Instead of going through the steps of deductive logic, she takes the shortcuts of natural reasoning.

> Johnny looks just as upset when he leaves school as he does when he comes in. There must be some problem at home that's keeping Johnny's mind off his work. I wonder what it could be. He's always recoiling when the kids get rough at horseplay, as if he's scared of being touched, and he always has his shirt buttoned up and his sleeves rolled down. Maybe he's being abused. I'll have to try to get a look at his arms and his chest.

In this flow of thoughts, the teacher commits some logical errors. Implicit in her reasoning is the following syllogism:

> Children who have problems at home are upset at leaving school.
> Johnny is upset at leaving school.
> Therefore Johnny has problems at home.

As we saw in the last section, the conclusion is not logically valid because the first premise only deals with one reason for being upset when leaving school. There could be other reasons why children are upset at leaving school: the big bully on the street corner, unwillingness to part with a schoolmate, and so on. Nevertheless it is perfectly reasonable for the teacher to reach the conclusion that she has if she regards it as tentative, which she does. The same type of invalid syllogism is contained in the teacher's next thought:

> Children who are abused recoil from physical contact (and keep their bodies covered).
> Johnny recoils from physical contact (and keeps his body covered).
> Therefore Johnny is abused.

Although logically unsound, the conclusion makes sense.

Because the teacher has a wide range of experience with children and how they behave, she is quick to associate Johnny's learning difficulties with his mood when he comes to and goes from school and she suspects abuse as the cause rather than another syndrome, such as delayed development, neurological impairment, or anger of the parents and child at being forced to educate the child at school. Instead of systematic consideration of these other possibilities, the teacher immediately looks for evidence to confirm her hunch, which is the natural way to think.

Being free from the strict rules of formal logic gives natural reasoning many advantages, but it also presents some potential pitfalls. To make the most of your natural reasoning, you must guard against the following common thinking traps.

Overgeneralizing

The ability to generalize often provides a sound basis for intelligent action. If you see a news clip about a mad dog and the dog is foaming at the mouth, you will probably generalize from this that all foaming dogs are mad and make sure that you steer clear of them. In this instance your generalization is based not only on the case of the foaming mad dog, but also on the many non-foaming normal dogs you have seen. Suppose, however, that you see a news clip about a dangerous woman driver. Many people generalize from such an experience that women are dangerous drivers. In this instance you would be overgeneralizing. For such a generalization to be reasonable, you would have to have seen many dangerous women drivers or many bad accidents in which the drivers were women, as well as no women drivers who were safe drivers. To make meaningful generalizations, you need to consider more than one or two isolated incidents, as well as related information.

Confusing Correlation and Causality

Often when two events happen at the same time, or one occurs right after the other, people assume that one event is causing the other. Children tend to think this way, especially where their own behavior is concerned. Many children who in a moment of anger at a sibling wished the other child dead feel that they have caused a sibling's misfortune if it follows shortly after the hostile thought. Adults, too, fall prey to this kind of thinking. Because people frequently have the experience that a bus comes every time they light up a cigarette, some half-jokingly light up a cigarette in order to make the bus come sooner. Correlated events are not necessarily causally related. Because the number of storks in Denmark is correlated with the birth rate, we do not conclude that the storks are responsible, but laugh it off as a cute co-incidence. Sometimes, however, two correlated events do seem to us to have a relationship and we are then prone to conclude that one is the result of the other, although there is no evidence to sustain such a conclusion. Many assume that the correlation of IQ scores with race means that race determines how intelligent you are. Even though these factors are related, the correlation does not mean that one causes the other. The lower IQ scores of minority groups could be caused by the lack of adequate nutri-tion, stimulation, and schooling suffered by people in the lower socioeconomic levels. Similarly, because there is a higher rate of emotional disturbance among children of divorced parents than among children of married parents, this does not necessarily mean that divorce causes the emotional disturbance. There is also a lower rate of income among divorced parents; it may be that the financial pressure is the factor leading both to emotional disturbance and to divorce.

Relying on Context

There is a tendency to let the context unduly influence our judgments of the elements contained in it. Some shoppers, for instance, think they are getting a higher quality suit or dress if they buy it at an expensive boutique rather than at a discount store, even though the merchandise in question may be the same. Such thinking is limiting and inaccurate. Relying on context is less work than making independent evaluations, because you are borrowing thoughts and ideas already created for you by the context rather than developing your own, but when you can look at an idea or object outside of its usual context, you can evaluate it in a new light and be more productive in your thinking.

Exercise _____

Read the following quotation and try to evaluate it in an independent rather than context-dependent manner: On a piece of paper write down whether or not you agree with the statement and why. Also write down whether you think the statement supports or contradicts the ideals of American democracy. Finish this exercise before reading on.

> This country, with its institutions, belongs to the people who inhabit it. Whenever they grow weary of the existing government, they can exercise their constitutional right of amending it, or their revolutionary right to dismember or overthrow it.
>
> —Karl Marx

_____

A lot of people who read the above statement disagree with it strongly because they are opposed to the Communistic ideas of Karl Marx, and/or to revolutions. They feel Marx's ideas threaten the American way of life. Some people agree with the statement because they believe, even if Communists think so too, that governments should bend to the will of the citizenry or be removed, and that this represents the American way. What was your answer? Do you agree or disagree with the statement? Do you believe it represents the American way or is opposed to the

American way? Actually, the statement above was not made by
Karl Marx, but by Abraham Lincoln. Does that make you change
your mind? Read it over again and think for a minute. Are you
letting yourself be influenced by the context established by the
presumed author, rather than by the statement? No matter who
wrote the statement, it expresses the foundations of our system of
government and our historical right to the revolutionary war of
independence.

To sum up, do not let yourself rely on the context; evaluate
things by their particular characteristics.

Relying on Authority

Often we take the word of an authority on important issues
instead of doing our own thinking, in the mistaken belief that
the authority must know better than we do. Many people, for
example, think that they should not take a position on a nuclear
freeze but leave that to the experts to decide. True, authorities
often have more information than we do, but they are prey to the
same thinking traps that we are. Accept an argument from
someone else only if it makes sense to you and not just on the
basis that it comes from an authority. At the trial of John
Hinckley, the man who shot President Reagan, as many authorities on psychiatry testified that Hinckley was sane as testified
that he was insane. Ultimately, the jury had to weigh the so-
called expert testimony and make its own decision. Similarly, try
not to rely on a physician's recommendation for surgery, a
stockbroker's recommendation to buy shares, or any other expert
opinion unless you have weighed that opinion and it is reasonable to you.

Relying on Statistics

Statistics have come to be another type of authority for us. If
somebody comes up with a figure, we tend to take that as
definitive; but figures can lie too. To take one instance, a lot of
data comes to us in the form of survey statistics, but the results of
many surveys are biased because they may be poorly conceived
and conducted among unrepresentative samples. If you ask a
respondent, "What is wrong with socialized medicine?" you will
get back critical statements, which you might be tempted to
interpret as indicating that people are opposed to socialized

medicine. If you ask instead, "What are some of the advantages and disadvantages of socialized medicine?" you may get an entirely different response from the same person and if you ask, "How do you feel about socialized medicine?" you might obtain a still different point of view. If you interview physicians for a survey on socialized medicine, you are going to get different statistics than if you interview uninsured patients in hospitals. Statistics reveal only part of the picture and can be manipulated either consciously or unconsciously to project a certain point of view. Take care when relying on statistics, especially on controversial issues. Be sure that you understand how the figures were obtained.

Relying on Consensus

It may be reassuring to know that a lot of other people have the same idea you do, but that is no guarantee that your idea makes sense. Despite common beliefs of the past, for example, your face will not break out in pimples if you masturbate, and evil will not befall you if a black cat crosses your path. And, despite common beliefs of the present, your intelligence is not set at birth and your IQ scores can be raised through coaching. Popular opinion is not necessarily informed opinion, so do not look to it to guide your thinking.

Relying on Narrow Definitions

Some people tend to view things in a narrowly defined way, while others define things flexibly. An inflexible person who needed to knock a nail into the wall would go looking for a hammer and, lacking one, would probably wait to borrow one from a neighbor. Another person might bang the nail in with a brick, wrench, or any other heavy object near at hand. One of our favorite examples of flexibility in definition occurs in the movie *Gone with the Wind*. Do you remember the scene in which Scarlett O'Hara needs a new dress and has no money to buy fabric? She rips the old velvet drapes off the wall and has them sewn into a sumptuous gown. The other characters, who adopt fixed definitions, look at the drapes and see drapes. Scarlett does not see just drapes, but yards of material hanging on the window.

Many food packagers get around consumers' tendency to stay locked into definitions by redefining foods and thereby getting you to buy more of their product. Mayonnaise labels, for example, offer recipes that let you use the product as a substitute for shortening in baking cakes and cereal boxes give you recipes for using cereal instead of flour when making cookies. The freer you are at redefining objects to suit your needs, the more adept you can be at problem-solving.

Thinking in Either-Or Terms

We have a tendency to think in terms of extreme alternatives rather than to consider more loosely defined possibilities. The more ambiguous things are, the more difficult it becomes to make decisions, which is one reason we look for clear-cut answers. Most things, however, are not simply black or white and we have to learn how to deal with the gray areas. Even such seemingly clear differences as dead or alive turn out to be difficult to discriminate. When life ends is now accepted as open to varying interpretations. Of course, most of us do not ordinarily have to get involved in decisions of life or death, but we do face various situations where either-or thinking can impede intelligent evaluation. In making decisions about marital separation, for example, where extreme positions are typically taken because of emotional pressures, there is rarely one mate who is right and one who is wrong; fault can be found on both sides. In evaluating political candidates, there is usually not one who is qualified and one who is unqualified, but more often two who are partially qualified. Most things and most people are not one-dimensional, but a composite of good and bad, and each positive quality has its negative aspect. To think intelligently we must often consider degrees rather than settle on absolutes.

Ignoring Details

To derive meaning from diverse information, we try to fit it into unified concepts. In the process, there is often a tendency to gloss over details. At the extreme, this can lead to faulty concepts that ignore vital facts. Even when this does not occur, the concept that loses detail loses much of its richness and meaning. This is illustrated by two descriptions we have heard of the United States in relation to its ethnic composition. The usual description takes a nonspecific, general point of view: "The United States is like a melting pot." The other description emphasizes

the component parts: "The United States is like a tossed salad."
One concept reduces the individual differences on which our
culture is based, the other preserves them. Try not to lose sight of
the particular in creating a meaningful whole, but put together
larger units that maintain the individuality of their parts.

CREATIVE THINKING

Creative thinking is the ability to produce new and unique ideas.
Sometimes creative thoughts consist of a rearrangement of facts
and ideas in a new configuration, and sometimes creative thoughts
consist of grasping patterns and order where none existed before.

One of the longstanding myths about creative thinking is that
it occurs spontaneously, the result of a flash of insight rather
than of applied rational thought. This conception came to us
from creative people who got their insights suddenly and, perhaps, unexpectedly through an "Aha" experience. Archimedes
steps into the bathtub, has a sudden flash of insight about the
principles of water displacement, and runs through the streets
shouting "Eureka!" Coleridge has an opium reverie and the
lines of "Kubla Khan" just come to him. Kekule has a dream and
sees how the atoms of the benzene ring fit together. Even our
cartoons illustrate the concept of creative thinking by means of
an electric bulb, which suddenly lights up over the character
who has a new idea.

It is true that creative thoughts often register at moments
when we do not make conscious effort, but they only come to the
mind that is already prepared. The flash of insight is the culmi-
nation of a process of concentrated thought. As D. N. Perkins
suggests in *The Mind's Best Work*, the *Aha* is the elation one
experiences when the pieces of a problem with which one has
been struggling finally fall into place. Creative thought, according to several theories, involves a number of stages. Perhaps
the most widely agreed on are those described by Graham Wallas
in 1926. First is the preparatory phase, also called the acquisition
stage or seeding the mind with information. The more you
immerse yourself in a topic, and the more data you plug into
your mind and comprehend, the greater the possibilities for
discovering new combinations and relationships. As Louis
Pasteur observed, "Chance favors the prepared mind."

The second phase of creative thought is incubation. During incubation you ponder the problem and what you already know, sometimes in bouts of concentrated thought, sometimes in fleeting review, and sometimes in what is called preconscious thought. Incubation gives you time to integrate the new input with stored information and allows your ideas to intermix and connect. This process leads to illumination, the *Aha* stage, at which point the kaleidoscopic array of ideas in your mind suddenly coalesces into a new pattern. Incubation and illumination are also called the transformation stage, in which old ideas are transformed into new concepts. There still is one more stage to creative thought—the verification process. An idea, to be truly creative, must work. Once formulated it has to be tested according to some standard. Sometimes our brilliant thoughts do not seem so well-conceived after a bit more reflection and it is necessary to put them back in the incubator.

To increase your efficiency during the preparation phase, the best procedure, obviously, is to expose yourself to as much information as you can. Einstein had to know math and physics before he could create the theory of relativity; Kekule had to understand atomic structure before he could solve the riddle of the benzene ring; and Leonardo da Vinci had to study anatomy before he could create his brilliant drawings of the human body.

To increase your efficiency during the incubation and illumination phases, there are a variety of approaches to use. Of utmost importance are motivation and hard work. As we will discuss in the chapter on emotions, exceptional mental achievement is associated with determination and dedication. Another approach to increasing illumination is to develop your visualization ability. One of the distinctive aspects of illumination is that it most often occurs in a visual form. Einstein reported that he visualized all the problems on which he worked and also visualized the solutions. Kekule solved the riddle of the benzene ring when he saw the atoms whirling and then saw the tail end of the chain attaching itself to the head, "like a snake eating its tail." Elias Howe's solution to the sewing machine came through a visual image of a needle with the eye in the point. Some suggestions for visualizing have been offered in a previous section of this chapter.

An important aid to creative transformation is putting yourself in a frame of mind that allows for the freer interplay of ideas. One of the reasons creative ideas seem to come to us effortlessly is that they often appear when we are not conscious of thinking, as when dreaming and daydreaming or at times of rest and relaxation. At these moments thought is not really suspended but of a different order. Often when we think deliberately we are more restrictive of the types of ideas we will allow and the rational demands we place on them. When we think in more relaxed states we give freer reign to our thoughts and imagination and let them wander as they will. The recent interest in altered states of consciousness is precisely that it is possible through such states to free yourself for more creative thinking. We will discuss this topic more fully in the chapter "Hidden Powers of the Mind," along with directions for getting in touch with these different aspects of consciousness.

Brainstorming and synectics are two techniques that have been employed for encouraging greater freedom of thinking and intermixing of ideas. Brainstorming is a group approach to problem-solving developed by an advertising executive, Alex Osborn, in which people sit down together and share their far-out thoughts, the assumption being that one idea will stimulate another. A similar approach, developed by William Gordon and called *synectics*, puts a group of experts together representing different fields for the purpose of evoking far-out thoughts, no matter how impossible, primarily by use of analogies. First the experts are asked to study the problem in detail, and then to come up with solutions that, even though wild, may prove useful. The idea is to first "make the strange familiar," then to "make the familiar strange."

In addition to the myth about the spontaneous occurrence of creative ideas, there is another myth to dispel. This one, like the intelligence myth, is that creativity is bestowed on some people but not others. Accordingly, there is a growing body of creativity tests that purportedly measure creativity, as distinct from intelligence. That creativity is viewed as a separate entity, rather than as a vital aspect of intelligence, is another reflection of the paucity of the standard concept of intelligence and the IQ.

Below are some typical items included on creativity tests:

Universal uses. Subjects are asked to give unusual uses for a common object such as a brick. A creative answer, recorded by J. P. Guilford, who designed this test, was *bug-hider*: "Put the brick on the ground for a week, then pick it up and look at the bugs hiding under it."

Impossible situations. Subjects are asked to imagine an impossible situation and its consequences, such as what would happen if a person could be invisible at will.

Incomplete figures. The subject is given an incomplete figure and asked to sketch it into a larger design that no one else will be apt to think of.

Original stories. Subjects are asked to write a story on a specific topic, such as "The lion that doesn't roar" or "The monkey that can fly."

Original drawings. In a variation on the above theme, subjects are asked to draw a picture illustrating a title, such as "Playing Tag in the School Yard." An original response, according to Jacob Getzels and Philip Jackson who created this task, was a drawing of a school with broken windows and graffiti reading, "Down with the Faculty," and "I hate children," and a note explaining, "It is the ghosts who are playing tag."

Remote associations. This test, developed by S. Mednick, asks the subject to think of a word that connects three given words. For example the words *rat, blue,* and *cottage* can be connected by the word *cheese.*

Although testing creativity has little validity because creativity cannot be measured or turned on at will, you can try to develop your own creative flow by practicing specific exercises modeled after the types of items used on creativity tests.

Exercise

Below are a variety of exercises in creative thinking. Before working on a problem, relax, make yourself comfortable, and give yourself a quiet place to sit without loud noises and distractions. As you think about the problems, let your imagination run wild. Do not censor your ideas, but let them flow. Try to visualize all your thoughts as vividly as possible—try to see them, smell them, hear them, and touch them.

- Imagine some new animals in the evolutionary tree that would be suited to new ecological conditions.

- Make up new names to fit the personalities of your friends and acquaintances, along the lines of Dickens's Mr. Scrooge.

- Design your dream-house for different locations. What is the ideal vacation beach house, ideal town house, and so on.

- Create a flag for the different countries of the world that would pictorially suggest some important aspect of the country, to replace the customary stripes, circles, and stars.

- Suppose you are a dealer in some basic material—wood, paper, metal, leather, plastics, glass—and want to increase your sales. What new uses can you promote for your material? Then turn the problem around: you are a manufacturer of clothing or chairs, household utensils and so on. What new materials and designs can you make to offer the public?

- Imagine the consequences of unusual situations. What if the earth's orbit around the sun grew progressively smaller so that each year the average temperature on earth would increase several degrees. Think of many consequences: physical, economic, psychological, and so on.

Basic to creative thinking is your attitude towards new ideas. The stereotype of the mad genius suggests that we tend to think of people who generate unusual ideas as a little crazy. This is because their ideas are usually a little wild and it is this quality that makes their thinking creative. To be more creative, don't be afraid of crazy ideas. Try not to prejudge your thoughts, and try to generate a lot more ideas than you can use. Attack problems with enthusiasm; if you don't get where you want right away, don't stop but start over. You will be creative if you feel you are creative.

Exercise

Take a problem that is important to you that you have been unable to solve. Try to work on it through all the creative stages. First, immerse yourself in the problem and find out all you can about it— read up on it, ask others about their experiences with it, and so on. Then, let the problem sit with you for a week or so, giving it a chance to incubate. After a while, put your mind to it more actively, trying to develop analogies, to visualize the problem, to let your imagination roam. If you come up with any new solutions, be sure to test them out.

Part of the difficulty in thinking in new and creative ways is that we are bogged down in old ways of thinking. As Edward de Bono has described it, people tend to think vertically, that is, to keep digging down deeper to solve a problem instead of thinking laterally by moving off to another spot and digging a new hole. In vertical thinking you choose the most promising approach and follow it as far as it can go; in lateral thinking you acknowledge the most likely approach but deliberately set out to find alternatives. Ultimately the difference between creative and noncreative thinking is your ability to break through the old mental sets that restrict your thinking to familiar patterns. The next chapter explores how you can accomplish that.

THE POWER
OF NEGATIVE THINKING

Positive thinking has become synonymous in our vocabulary with *successful thinking* and is taken for granted as a good thing. Few people realize, however, that positive thinking is basically not thinking at all. Positive thinking is an affirmation of past experiences: it says "yes" to accumulated knowledge and what has already been thought. As such, positive thinking is unoriginal, leading to conformity to popularly held ideas. Genuine thinking, by contrast, occurs not by accepting yesterday's conclusions, but by going beyond the old and developing the new. Genuine thinking is negative thinking: it says "no" to outworn ideas and takes nothing for granted. When you use negative thinking, you free yourself from automatic thinking patterns and evaluate things for yourself. While positive thinking is a passive process that blunts your intelligence, negative thinking is an active process that stimulates your intelligence.

Because the world is such a complicated place, we try to get along in it by depending on other people's knowledge and experience rather than using our own heads. This makes us mentally lazy and less alert. We tend to forget that the information we absorb and assumptions we take for granted may not be valid and may actually keep us from approaching problems intelligently. We can look back at human history and smile indulgently at the silly thoughts people used to have—that praying to the rain god would make the showers come or that sailing off towards the horizon would make you fall off the earth—but just as these commonly accepted theories of yesterday caused people to behave in nonintelligent ways, the same process operates today. To think intelligently means to stop and look carefully at all the ideas and so-called facts you take for granted and to start questioning things critically.

Instead of saying to yourself, "This must be so because I read it in the paper or saw it in a book, heard it on the radio, learned it from my teacher," ask: "Is this true? What evidence has been presented? Is there anything in my experience that contradicts this? Can I explain this a better way?" To be more intelligent, you have to free yourself from stereotyped ways of thinking and think for yourself. Instead of lulling you into following other people, negative thinking puts you ahead of the pack.

NEGATIVE THINKERS
ARE CREATIVE THINKERS

All the people who have made a major contribution to the world's knowledge have been negative thinkers and all were originally penalized for their audacity in questioning established ways of thinking. For example, Galileo, who experimentally confirmed the fact that the sun and not the earth is the center of the universe, was labeled a heretic and forced to recant his discoveries by the Inquisition. Columbus was derided for being negative enough to think that the earth was round when everyone accepted the idea that it was flat. Robert Fulton's steamboat was called "Fulton's Folly" because his contemporaries thought the idea so ridiculous. Samuel Morse had a hard time getting the telegraph patented and Congress refused to buy his invention, expecting that it would not be worth the money. Alexander Graham Bell had a similar experience with his telephone. He gave successful demonstrations, but most people thought the instrument was too silly to use. Thomas Edison was fired from his job as telegrapher because he spent part of his time at work inventing a gadget that recorded messages automatically regardless of the speed at which they were sent, and the company thought he was wasting his time and their money.

The list of negative thinkers goes on and on into our own time. Freud was ostracized by the medical profession in Vienna for suggesting that unconscious thoughts lay behind physical symptoms and that people had a lot of sexual urges that they were repressing. Einstein's negative thinking initially kept him from getting the grades necessary for acceptance to graduate school; later, his thesis on relativity was turned down by his dissertation committee. And so it goes. What first sounds ridiculous often turns out to be a new discovery. The negative thinkers who challenge the old are free to discover the new.

Let's take a look at how a creative thinker actually solved a problem. Edward Jenner hit upon the idea of the smallpox vaccine by negative thinking. In his day, there was no known remedy for smallpox. However, some people who were exposed to the disease did not catch it. Positive thinking focused on the obvious question: Why do people get smallpox? Edward Jenner, however, asked the opposite question: Why don't people get smallpox? By studying people who did not get the disease, even though exposed to it, Jenner discovered his immunization technique. He found that milkmaids, who worked with cows, never caught smallpox. The reason was they caught cowpox, which provided them with an immunity to the more serious disease. Jenner's innoculation against smallpox was based on the immunizing properties of cowpox. The physicians of Jenner's day violently opposed his vaccination.

You may be thinking that you'll never be an Edward Jenner, or an Edison, or an Einstein, but that too is an example of how positive thinking limits you. We assume that some people are brilliant and have what it takes, but that the rest of us can never reach such heights. Probably nobody, including you, suspects you might be a genius, but then nobody suspected that the shaggy-haired man who worked as an examiner in the Zurich patent office would win a Nobel prize for formulating the theory of relativity. Brilliant thoughts and new ideas can occur to anyone who takes the trouble to turn old ideas upside down, inside out, and round about. When you get rid of your positive thinking habits, your mind too can take off in new, creative directions.

BLOCKS TO NEGATIVE THINKING

You may not realize it, but you are a born negative thinker. As children, our minds are still unconditioned and we spontaneously test everything out for ourselves. Taking apart the clock to see what makes it tick is a common example of negative thinking at work. So is the *why* stage that children go through with its endless stream of questions: "Why is there grass, why is it green, why isn't the sky green too, why can birds fly, why can't I fly, why, why, why?" Before long, we are discouraged from negative thinking. Children learn to inhibit their natural questioning attitude because the surrounding adults start to express annoyance at the barrage of *whys.* Hearing questions from children makes people anxious because, among other things, it highlights their own intellectual gaps. How many parents know why the grass is green or, more importantly, ever think to ask? The mother who feels pestered says, "Stop asking mommy so many questions and just do what I say." The teacher who feels threatened by questions not included in the syllabus says, "Stop disrupting the class and just make sure you know today's lesson because I'm going to test you on it tomorrow." Children quickly learn that adults are not interested in how children think but in how well they can absorb what they are told. In fact, children who raise too many questions and think for themselves are often scolded and labeled as wise guys or smart alecks. Negative thinking becomes foreign to us not because it is inherently difficult, but because we are conned into positive thinking by our need to belong. Even intelligence tests, as a later chapter shows, reward people who accept what they are told and penalize those who think for themselves.

When people are dissuaded from having unique thoughts, they start to mistrust their own thinking. Just how far this tendency to mistrust one's own thinking ability can go is demonstrated in an ingenious experiment that we already referred to in the chapter on perception. People were asked to participate in a study on judging comparative lengths. The experimenter showed pairs of sticks of different lengths and asked subjects to say which was the longer. The judgments were obtained in a group setting in which, unknown to the subjects, the other members were actually confederates of the experimenter and had been instructed to make incorrect judgments. What happened was that a large percentage of people were not able to make accurate judgments when the confederates in the room gave incorrect judgments. Instead, they modified their answers to fall in line with group opinion. Some negative thinkers held firm and consistently gave correct answers no matter how much the group tried to pressure them into wrong answers, but most subjects were swayed. Interviews after the experiment revealed that a few subjects knew they were giving wrong answers and did not want to stand out in the group, but most gave wrong answers because they began to mistrust their own judgment and would not believe their own eyes!

CLEARING YOUR MIND
FOR NEGATIVE THINKING

To regain your ability to think negatively, you have to first clear your mind of the positive thinking habits that get in your way. Without realizing it, most people are stuck in rigid ways of thinking, which block their intelligence. They automatically use old thinking habits to solve new problems. The following exercises will demonstrate to you how easy it is to develop unproductive mental sets. Practicing on these problems will also illustrate the traps to avoid and help awaken your intelligence.

Exercise

The Water Jar

This series of problems is adapted from those developed by the psychologist Abraham Luchins. Complete the problems in sequence and write down your solution to each problem on a piece of paper. The problems require you to measure out a specified amount of water by transferring water from different-sized jars.

Problem 1: There are two empty jars: a 39-quart jar and a 4-quart jar, and an unlimited supply of water. The problem is to measure out 31 quarts of water using these jars.

Work it out with paper and pencil and write down your steps. If you're stuck, here is the solution: fill the 39-quart jar and then from this fill the 4-quart jar. This leaves 35 quarts in the big jar. Dump the water in the 4-quart jar and fill it again from the big jar. This leaves 31 quarts in the big jar, and the problem is solved (big jar minus small jar twice). Now try the next problem.

Problem 2: There are three different-sized jars: 31 quarts, 61 quarts, and 4 quarts. The problem is to measure out 22 quarts of water using these jars.

Try working it out with paper and pencil. If you get stuck, check the solution, but only after you have tried to work it out on your own. The solution: Fill the 61-quart jar and then, from this jar, fill the 31-quart jar one time and the 4-quart jar twice. Then 22 quarts of water remain in the 61-quart jar (big jar minus medium jar minus small jar twice). From now on, you're on your own. Do the remaining problems without stopping, writing down your solutions as you go along. Do not check the answers until you have finished all the problems.

Problem 3: There are 3 jars: 30 quarts, 40 quarts, and 3 quarts. Obtain 4 quarts of water.

Problem 4: There are 3 jars: 14 quarts, 59 quarts, and 10 quarts. Obtain 25 quarts of water.

Problem 5: There are 3 jars: 9 quarts, 42 quarts, and 6 quarts. Obtain 21 quarts of water.

Problem 6: There are 3 jars: 18 quarts, 43 quarts, and 10 quarts. Obtain 5 quarts of water.

Problem 7: There are 3 jars: 17 quarts, 40 quarts, and 6 quarts. Obtain 11 quarts of water.

Problem 8: There are 3 jars: 11 quarts, 25 quarts, and 3 quarts. Obtain 8 quarts of water.

Problem 9: There are 3 jars: 10 quarts, 23 quarts, and 3 quarts. Obtain 7 quarts of water.

Problem 10: There are 3 jars: 11 quarts, 27 quarts, and 5 quarts. Obtain 6 quarts of water.

What method did you use for solving the problems? If you're like most people, you solved them all the same way: big jar minus medium jar minus small jar twice. This is a correct solution, but it is not the most intelligent solution. Take another look at problems 7, 8, 9 and 10. There is an easier way to solve them. Try to figure it out and write it down. You can solve the last four problems in one step: medium jar minus the small jar.

Most people get into the habit of thinking a certain way and then stick to it even when it isn't useful any more. If you solved all the problems by the long method instead of switching to the short method, you had firsthand experience of how your thinking can get stuck in a rut. Now stay on your toes for the next exercise and think negatively. Don't let your mind get set in an automatic pattern.

Exercise _____

Hidden Words

In this series of problems, also adapted from Luchins, your task is to find the four- or five-letter word hidden in the string of letters, without changing the order of the letters. Copy over the problem on a sheet of paper, and then try to solve the problem. When you work these problems out, keep a written record of what you do.

Problem 1: What four- or five-letter word is hidden in this series of letters?

M T A U R S E

The answer is MARE. Now go on to the next problem.

Problem 2: What four- or five-letter word is hidden in this series of letters?

G Z O Q A R T

Having trouble figuring it out? The answer is GOAT. Now find the hidden four- or five-letter word in each series in problems 3 through 12.

Problem 3: B O U F L M L

Problem 4: D Z E P E W R

Problem 5: M D U R L I E

Problem 6: W I O R L Z F

Problem 7: B X E S A U R

Problem 8: T K I N G R E V R

Problem 9: H N O P R A S H E

Problem 10: G U O M O S S L E

Problem 11: C W A R M B E I L

Problem 12: M D O N U T Z G E

Let's check your answers. Yes, there is a solution that you can use on all but Problem 12: just cross out every other letter and you end up with the name of an animal. But this solution doesn't work with Problem 12, because then you end with MOUZE, which is not a real word. If you couldn't solve Problem 12, look again. Inside Problem 12 is a word with all the letters next to each other: DONUT. If you ended up with the names of animals on Problems 8, 9, 10, and 11 (TIGER, HORSE, GOOSE, CAMEL) you got correct answers, but you did not get the most intelligent answer. The most intelligent answer is the simple answer. Just like Problem 12, Problems 8, 9, 10, and 11 each contains a complete word directly in it: KING, RASH, MOSS, WARM. If you did not see these words, it is because you got stuck in one of two mental sets: either you were automatically checking off every other letter without looking for simpler solutions, or you were taking it for granted that every hidden word had to be the name of an animal. If you didn't get stuck, you're already thinking intelligently.

In these two exercises there was a long solution and a short solution. The sequence of problems was designed to let your mind develop a pattern of thinking, which then became hard to break. We wanted to show you how the process works and how you can think correctly without necessarily thinking intelligently. Now that you have seen how easy it is to fall into unproductive mental sets, it should make you more alert the next time you have a problem to solve.

If you're thinking that these problems were tricks and do not represent ordinary thinking situations, that is not exactly so. Admittedly, they were set up for you to slip into automatic thinking, but that is what happens in everyday life situations as well. Without being aware of it, you have been trained to think in automatic ways that make it more difficult for you to think intelligently and to be alert to new possibilities. For example, because you were taught to count in the decimal system, where everything is based on tens, it is much harder for you to learn how to use a numerical system based on twelve, which is fundamentally simpler. Children who learn the new math in school can switch around from one base system to another without any trouble, but adults get stuck because they have become set in their way of thinking. For the same reason, learning a new language or any other skill is easier when you do it at a young age before your thinking becomes rigid. That is one of the reasons why most creative discoveries are made by people in their twenties and thirties.

HOW TO USE NEGATIVE THINKING TO SOLVE PROBLEMS

One of the best illustrations of negative thinking applied to problem-solving is found in the area of puzzles, brainteasers, riddles, and murder mysteries. The fascination of these thinking exercises lies in their unique solutions, which require negative thinking. Detective stories usually provide a set of clues making us suspect the wrong person of the crime; the murderer turns out to be the character you have forgotten about. Similarly, most riddles stump us if we think positively and get programmed in a set way of thinking, but can easily be solved if we think negatively. For example:

> What name was given to the first satellite to go around the earth?
>
> (Hint: positive thinking directs your attention to man-made satellites, while negative thinking frees you to answer the question.)

Answer: the moon.

How can you close this book without touching it?

(Hint: positive thinking programs you to think of different physical manipulations you can make; negative thinking tells you to try a new approach.)

Answer: Let someone else do it for you.

The solutions to most riddles and other brainteasers are usually quite simple, but unexpected. Negative thinking helps you approach such problems intelligently by freeing you from mental sets and opening up your mind to new and unusual solutions.

Exercise

Take a look now at some thinking problems. In trying to solve them, don't think the way the problem programs you, but think negatively.

The Mouse: A girl went to feed her pet mouse in the morning and found it alive and well but with its rear end sticking out of the cage, stuck between the bars. She was confused and couldn't figure out how that happened. Although she knew her mouse had tried to escape before, it never moved backward before. What do you think happened?

Solution: The girl assumed her mouse was trying to get out of the cage and got stuck. What really happened was that the mouse was trying to get back into its cage! The mouse had already escaped, scrambled up a bite to eat in the kitchen, and on its way back in fattened condition, had been unable to make it through the bars.

Surgeon: A young man was brought to a hospital after being injured in an automobile accident. The emergency room physician examined him and decided that surgery was required to save his life. The surgeon was called but upon seeing the patient exclaimed, "Oh no. I can't operate on him. He's my son." This was so, but the surgeon was not the young man's father. How can you resolve this seeming contradiction?

Solution: Positive thinking takes it for granted that the surgeon is a man. Negative thinking points in the opposite direction: why can't the surgeon be a woman? If the surgeon is a woman, she can be a parent without being a father.

Architect: How can an architect build a house in the form of a cube and have windows in every wall that all face south?

Solution: The way the problem is stated it leads you to expect that the solution is a structural one of how the house is built. Turn the problem around and ask yourself a different question. The problem tells you how to build the house—a cube with windows in each wall. You have to ask yourself *where* to build the house. At what point on the earth's surface can you turn around 360 degrees and keep looking south? That's right—build the house at the North Pole.

If negative thinking were only good for solving riddles and puzzles, it would be lots of fun, but not very practical. Negative thinking, however, can be applied to your day-to-day problems for fun *and* profit. Because it keeps you a step ahead of what others are thinking, negative thinking has proven particularly advantageous in business and investing. If you look at some of the great money-making ideas, you will find that they arose from negative thinking. Thomas Adams, of Chiclet fame, made a fortune on chewing gum because he gave it away when he couldn't sell it. Shopkeepers who did not want to carry his product did consent to give a piece away free with each store purchase. In this way Adams got people to try the gum and soon they started coming back to buy it. The inventors of the pet rock made a fortune selling, for two dollars and up, an ordinary rock packed in a box with a sheet of instructions for its care and feeding. They were successful because they would not accept the common assumption that you must offer customers something of value. The t-shirt craze enabled businesses to make double money by raking in profits on the t-shirts as well as getting free advertising. How many people wearing a t-shirt with a sales message on it are aware that they have paid for the privilege of advertising someone else's product and increasing someone else's profits?

On Wall Street, too, negative thinking can bring financial rewards. People who follow popular investment trends usually end up by losing money instead of making it. One striking illustration of this is the recent gold story. All through the late 1960s and early 1970s, established investment firms were advising people to put their money into stocks and bonds, while a few mavericks were urging people to buy gold instead. The popular view was that gold had no future because of the government's policy of holding the price down. Negative thinkers foresaw that the price of gold had to rise in an inflationary economy and that the government did not have the power to control it in world markets. Although the gold bugs were ridiculed, they made big profits when gold rose from $35 to $850 an ounce, while the majority of people lost money staying in conventional invest-ments. When gold caught on at high prices, negative thinking (the Wall Street term is *contrary opinion*) helped smart investors sell out before its downswing in response to temporary monetary restraint policies. Those who followed the popular view were caught on both the up and down swings.

Similarly, in real estate investments, negative thinking directs you towards buying what others don't want. Those big so-called white elephant homes, for example, that everyone shies away from can be one of the best real estate investments available. Large houses on large tracts of land usually sell for propor-tionately less because most people don't know what to do with such big places. In addition to leaving sufficient space for private living quarters, they can often take on special value when con-verted to condominium apartments, executive meeting centers, or restaurants. A white elephant can be a golden goose if you look at it from a negative point of view. Not too long ago in New York City a few negative thinkers got the idea of renting loft space in old warehouses. The space was vast and the rent was cheap because the buildings offered few conveniences. With the money saved from the rent, many of these lofts were converted into elegant living spaces. Now they are the craze in New York and have become very expensive. Because everybody wants one, now is not a good time, from a financial point of view, to rent one.

Intelligent and successful living requires that you approach personal life as well as your business life in a critical way, rather than just taking it for granted. When considering your health, your relationships, your children, or any other aspect of your life, negative thinking can help you stay on top of things.

Exercise

Let's look at some actual problem situations that people like you have faced, and see how negative thinking provided creative solutions. In trying to solve these problems remember: Do not take anything for granted; make sure you test out all your assumptions; avoid getting stuck in set ways of thinking; rephrase the questions you are trying to solve in a new form.

Bedtime: A seven-year-old girl was giving her parents a hard time about going to bed at night, making a fuss at the appointed bedtime and demanding that she be allowed to stay up just as late as her mother and father. What would you do in this situation? The usual way of handling this type of bedtime resistance is to discipline the child for misbehaving and to insist on obedience. Negative thinking suggested that instead of punishing the child for the annoying behavior, that the parents motivate the child to want to behave more appropriately. The parents made a deal with their daughter: they told her that they would consent to her going to bed when they did if she was ready to maintain their hours on a consistent schedule. On the first evening the girl was delighted to stay up until her parents went to bed around 11:30 P.M. On the second night she fell asleep in front of the TV set at 9 P.M., whereupon she was awakened and kept awake until her parents retired. On the third night the girl asked to go back to her own bedtime hour, and the problem was solved.

Ethnic Origins: A student applying to professional school was miffed that recent legislation provided less stringent admissions standards for minority persons but excluded him from participating in the program. What could he do? Thinking negatively, the student came up with the ingenious solution of having his name legally changed to a Spanish rendering of his own. He then had himself reclassified as "Hispanic," and became eligible for the affirmative action program. When minority groups protested that he was not genuinely Hispanic, he countered that he spoke a fluent Spanish, had lived in Puerto Rico for many years, and had a Spanish grandmother. Thus in terms of language group, cultural heritage, and ethnic origin, he was fully qualified within the law.

Part-Time Parents: A divorced couple with joint custody of their two children of eight and ten years were having difficulty working out a suitable plan for child care. They tried different arrangements: the children staying with one parent during the week and the other one on weekends, alternately staying at the mother's house one week and at the father's the next, and switching from one parent's home to the other's after a month's interval. The children were angry at both parents, resentful of the continual moving back and forth, and found it hard to keep up with schoolwork and meet with their friends. They asked to be allowed to stay put with only one parent, but both parents were unwilling to give up their time with the children. What would you have done? After much discussion, the parents agreed that it was better for the children to remain in one place. They reconciled this with the problem of joint custody by letting the children have a permanent place to live and having the parents alternate living at what became the children's home. In this way, the parents had separate but equal visiting rights and the children could lead happier lives.

Mail Order: A man sent a fifty-dollar check for a jacket to a mail-order firm. Although they cashed his check, they did not send the jacket. A lengthy correspondence ensued, during which the firm made all sorts of excuses: out of stock, computer error, shipment actually made, etc., but after many months the man still had no jacket and no fifty dollars. What could he do? Thinking negatively, the man reordered the jacket, but this time charged the order to his credit card. Sure enough, a jacket was delivered. As soon as it arrived, the man wrote to the firm canceling his order, stating that he no longer needed a second jacket since the first was just shipped. The credit company would not bill the man for the canceled order and his account was thereby settled.

Senior Citizens: The director of a senior citizens' program was trying to develop a plan for keeping senior citizens occupied in meaningful activities without spending any additional money. She could not hire recreational directors, or build new facilities, or invest in recreational supplies and equipment. What would you do in such a situation? As long as the director thought positively and asked "What can we do for our senior citizens?" she could not find a solution. When she looked at the problem negatively and turned the question around asking instead, "What can our senior citizens do for others?" a solution presented itself. By investigating to find out who needed help in the community, she found a shortage of teachers in day care and nursery facilities and put the senior citizens to work with the kids. The kids were delighted to have the extra attention and care from their new grandmas and grandpas and the older people were delighted to have the warm human contact and feel needed again. The plan was so successful that when the community built new day care centers, they attached a senior citizens' center as part of the unit.

These examples show you how negative thinking works and the wide variety of situations in which it can be used. You can raise your intelligence by applying negative thinking to the problems you face. At first you will have to make a conscious effort to look at things from a contrary perspective, but after a while it will come naturally. The more you use negative thinking, the more intelligent you will become and the more successful you will be in life.

RAISING YOUR IQ

Your IQ—or intelligence quotient—is supposed to be an objective measure of your intelligence. It is a measure, but it is not objective, and it is not a reflection of your intelligence. What it does measure is your ability to take IQ tests, which are based on skills you learn in school. Because these tests and others derived from them, such as college entrance tests, play a large role in determining your options in life, it is important that you do well on them. This chapter is designed to help you master the techniques of taking IQ tests and similar screening devices so that you can raise your scores.

Underlying intelligence tests are many faulty assumptions, the most basic of which is that your IQ, being a measure of your native intelligence, cannot be raised. By showing you how to raise your IQ, we also hope to dispel some of the myths surrounding these tests and expose some of the dangers in their use.

A SHORT HISTORY OF TESTING

The first attempt at intelligence testing was made approximately 100 years ago by Sir Francis Galton in England. Based on the theory that knowledge comes from the senses and that the most intelligent people are those with the most perfected senses, Galton's tests were designed to determine sensory acuity: keenness of hearing; reaction times to light, sound, and touch; ability to judge weight; etc. Galton was followed by an American psychologist named James Cattell, who coined the phrase *mental test* in 1890, and who added measures of time perception, color discrimination, accuracy of hand movement, and memory to Galton's measures of sensory function. These approaches were not successful, however, because they could not differentiate among people in regard to any other criteria of intellectual achievement.

In France, at about the same time, a psychologist named Alfred Binet was developing a test for the Ministry of Education that could identify children of low ability who needed special education. Binet believed that such testing must be based on the mental processes involved in intelligence rather than on sensory and motor functions. He assembled a series of tasks that related to everyday experience (for example, counting coins, drawing a square, identifying objects in terms of use, figuring out the meaning of a disarranged sentence) and involved such basic intellectual skills as comprehension and reasoning. He then determined which tasks could be performed by most children at any given age, and selected those tasks that showed the clearest age differences in the percent passing them. A four-year-old-level task would be placed on the test, for instance, if half the four-year-olds failed and half passed the task. Binet's test, which appeared in 1905, generated the concept of mental age (as opposed to chronological age), based on the child's ability to do tasks associated with the performance level of a certain age group. A few years after Binet's test appeared, William Stern, a German psychologist, suggested that it was more meaningful to divide the mental age (MA) by the chronological age (CA), rather than subtract it as Binet had done, since it is the relative disparity between the two that is significant. Stern called this relationship the IQ, and his formula was as follows:

$$\frac{MA}{CA} \times 100 = IQ.$$

The quotient was multiplied by 100 in order to eliminate decimals. An IQ of 100, where MA = CA, was considered normal.

Binet emphasized that his test did not measure intelligence and that it only reflected a child's capacity at a given moment. It was, in fact, because Binet believed in the possibility of increasing intellectual level that he felt it necessary to identify children who needed and could benefit from special education, which he dubbed *mental orthopedics*.

Although Binet stressed that intelligence was too complex to be reduced to a single score and cautioned against interpreting mental age as a measure of inherent intelligence, his warnings went unheeded. His test was imported into the United States by American psychologists, who translated it, popularized it, and perverted its intentions. They not only claimed that intelligence was inherited and that a person's IQ score was a reflection of that individual's fixed capacity, but they also maintained that the IQ should be used to determine a person's proper station in life. Whereas Binet wanted his test to be used to raise people's intellectual level, the early American adapters used it to limit people's opportunities.

Three men played important roles in this movement. Henry Goddard was the first to translate the Binet scale into English. He wanted to identify people below normal capacity so that they could be segregated and kept from immigrating into the country. Under his leadership, a research program was set up on Ellis Island to test the new arrivals. Because the test included many culture-loaded items which foreigners were unfamiliar with, the immigrants scored very low. His work helped to pave the way for later exclusionary immigration quotas.

The most influential American version of Binet's test was the one prepared by Lewis Terman of Stanford University, which became known as the Stanford-Binet. This revision was introduced in 1916. Unlike Goddard, Terman not only wanted to screen out so-called morons; he wanted to test everybody, hoping thereby to be able to assign all persons to their appropriate niche. Terman extolled the virtues of universal testing and envisaged a society in which IQs would serve as the entry key to various occupations.

A year after the introduction of the Stanford-Binet, Terman's dream of mass testing received a boost through the advent of World War I. Robert Yerkes, another American psychologist, sold the army on the idea of testing recruits in order to make personnel assignments and separate officer candidates from cannon fodder. Working with Terman, Goddard, and others, he developed the Army Alpha and Beta Tests, which could be administered to large groups of men in one hour's time, and a total of almost 2 million men were so tested. Like their predecessors, these tests were culturally biased and discriminated against the lower socioeconomic groups and recent immigrants.

Because of the publicity surrounding the army testing program, and its aura of scientific objectivity, many businesses and schools became interested in large-scale testing, an interest that was abetted by the advertisements of the testmakers. Terman, in conjunction with Yerkes and others, marketed the National Intelligence Tests for school children, which were touted as applying army testing methods to school needs. A host of competitors joined the field and soon a multimillion-dollar testing industry came into being.

The bias inherent in intelligence testing created a major social controversy in the 1920s, spearheaded by columnist Walter

Lippman; however, testing went ahead unimpeded. Criticism of the tests and their validity, coming mostly from the public sector, was discounted by the testmakers as the uninformed opinion of laypersons. Concern about the misuse of the tests surfaced again in the 1960s, when testing proliferated in the schools under the joint influence of federal funding and the appearance of automated test-scoring equipment. It was not until the 1970s, however, that popular concern over IQ testing peaked and brought with it a split among psychologists as well. In 1969, psychologist Arthur Jensen wrote an article for the *Harvard Educational Review* in which he attributed the obtained differences in IQ scores between whites and blacks to genetic factors. This view was echoed by Richard Herrnstein in an article in *Atlantic Monthly* in 1971, in which he argued that the demonstrated relationships between IQ and social class reflected a pattern of inherited stratification which would become more marked in the future, and that the nation should prepare for it rather than argue against it.

The battle over IQ testing continues. Volumes of papers are being written espousing both the view that intelligence is a measurable, inherited trait possessed in greater degree by the upper social strata and reflected in their higher IQ scores, and the view that intelligence is a fluid, undefinable quality with IQ scores reflecting social and educational advantages rather than inherited intellectual ability. Although the controversy is far from resolved, testing is still flourishing.

The growth of the testing industry rests on several factors. First, it enables schools, industry, and government agencies to deal with large numbers of people in a one- to two-hour testing period. Secondly, tests continue to have the aura of scientific objectivity, which gives them credence with the public. Thirdly, the relative inaccessibility of tests, test results, and testing procedures to public scrutiny enables the testing industry to protect the tests from challenges.

Interestingly, throughout it all, the Stanford-Binet remains the standard against which other tests have been measured. It is reasoned that since the Stanford-Binet measures intelligence (an unfounded statement), any test that correlates with it also measures intelligence (a compounded unfounded statement). The original Binet test, which its creator warned "does not permit the measure of intelligence," is thus used to give other tests their respectability as valid indicators of intelligence. The best use of

IQ tests is still as an aid in diagnosing learning problems, which was Binet's original intention, and not to classify the overall intellectual worth of people.

THE TESTING INDUSTRY

Every year since the introduction of the Stanford-Binet has brought new tests into the field. There are so many different tests now marketed for so many situations that mandate testing, that it is hard for anyone growing up in this country not to have taken a test at some time or other. In fact, it is estimated that many people take roughly ten standardized tests during the course of their schooling, while conservative estimates put the number at three. Whichever is the correct figure, the amount of tests given nationally has risen from 5 million annually in 1930 to 10 million in 1960 to 500 million in 1980. The Educational Testing Service, which gives approximately 8 million tests a year, or only about one-sixth of the national total, makes $94 million a year on its testing operation. Obviously, keeping you taking tests is big business.

Unlike other industries, which offer the customer a choice of whether to buy or not to buy, the testing industry provides no such options. IQ tests are built into the schooling process and test results are made a permanent part of the school records. Moreover, it is only recently that people are even able to obtain their scores on many of these tests. Before the Family Education Rights and Privacy Act was passed in 1974, many testers would not provide results, under the rationale that lay people would not know how to interpret them properly.

Because so many critical decisions about a person's life depend on test results, it is natural that people are concerned about how well they do on the tests they have to take. Thus, a corollary coaching industry has developed alongside of the testing industry. It is estimated that the coaching schools take in $60 million annually; and these schools concentrate only on college and professional admissions tests. The testing industry maintains that coaching is useless, a position they are bound to take since they claim that their tests measure innate intellectual aptitudes. Nevertheless, studies have shown that coaching can and does improve scores by a significant amount.

One of the most important benefits of coaching is to provide you with experience in test-taking. Research shows that people usually score higher on a second, alternate test than on the first test taken. Similarly, persons with prior experience in taking standardized tests do better than persons taking their first test. Familiarity with types of questions included on tests and with use of the answer booklets are other factors improving performance. Coaching also helps by supplementing educational gaps that the test-taker might have.

In addition to coaching schools, several books and popular articles have appeared that provide tips on how to take tests. Basically, they offer the reader familiarity with test-taking procedures and the specific types of questions one is likely to meet. These include Arthur Whimbey's *Intelligence Can Be Taught*, Bernard Feder's *The Complete Guide to Taking Tests*, the *Reader's Digest* piece "You Can Raise Your Child's IQ," and the Scholastic Aptitude Test (SAT), Graduate Record Examination (GRE), and other test preparatory booklets published by Barron's, Amsco, and other companies. This chapter includes pointers applicable to all tests, but if you know what test you have to take, we recommend that you look through the available booklets designed to coach you in that specific test.

VARIETIES OF TESTS

Intelligence tests come in a variety of forms. There are the paper-and-pencil tests that come in printed booklets, in which the test subject writes the answers or checks the multiple-choice alternatives. Paper-and-pencil tests can be administered with minimal supervision to one person or to many people at one time. Individual tests are administered on a one-to-one basis, with the examiner asking the questions and writing down the answers. Individual tests sometimes encompass puzzlelike tasks, which can not be performed on a group basis.

Most paper-and-pencil tests are timed to measure how quickly and efficiently you can perform. Many items on individual tests are also timed, but the one-to-one situation also allows for the inclusion of "power tests," which are untimed to determine the highest level of ability that can be achieved without pressure.

IQ tests vary on the types of items they contain. Most contain verbal items (vocabulary, verbal analogies, comprehension, and general information); some only nonverbal items (pattern completion, figural analogies, number series completion, figure series completions); some only performance items (jigsaw puzzle problems, block designs, mazes, copying designs); and some contain a variety of items from all these categories. Most paper-and-pencil tests yield one IQ score, but individual tests are often scored to yield both a *Verbal IQ* and a *Performance IQ*, as well as a *Full Scale IQ*. We will describe some typical items and how to work with them a little later on.

The most popularly used paper-and-pencil tests in the United States include the following: Otis Quick-Scoring Mental Ability Test, Pintner General Ability Tests, California Test of Mental Maturity, Lorge-Thorndike Intelligence Tests, Henmon-Nelson Tests of Mental Ability, and the Kuhlmann-Anderson Tests.

The two most popular individually administered tests are the Stanford-Binet Intelligence Scale and the Wechsler Intelligence Scales for adults (WAIS) and for children (WISC). Because the latter provide subscores for various mental functions that can be compared with each other, they are often used for diagnostic purposes as well as for determining overall IQ.

WHAT YOUR IQ MEANS

To understand what the IQ really tells us about a person, we have to look a little more closely at how IQ tests are constructed and scored. Today's IQ scores are no longer calculated on the basis of the MA to CA ratio. Instead, the raw score (or total number of items correct) is converted into an IQ score based on a comparison of a person's score with those in a standardized group. The standardization group is a sample of persons used to establish norms for the test, who are supposedly representative of the general population. If you obtain an IQ score of 100 it means that you scored higher than 50 percent of the people of your age in the standardization group, but not as high as the other 50 percent, making you average for your age. A score above 100 means you are above the average for your age, while a score below 100 means you are below the average. The testmakers assumed that intelligence does not increase past age sixteen, and the functions tapped by IQ tests do not show increases in ability much past that age. For this reason, the IQ score cannot be calculated on the basis of the MA to CA ratio for adults, because they would then all show a continual drop in their intelligence. Mental qualities that keep growing after age sixteen—knowledge, understanding, and wisdom—are not measured by IQ tests.

Because your IQ tells you where you stand in relation to your age group, your scores can go up and go down without this meaning that your abilities are increasing or decreasing. It is usual for people with lower IQs to show increases as they get older and for people with higher IQs to show decreases as they get older, just because the composition of their reference group changes. The IQ does not tell you about your absolute standing, but only where you are in relation to others.

Testmakers assume that intelligence is distributed among people in such a way that there are relatively few with low or high intelligence and many with average intelligence—and so each question must show a similar distribution of responses, otherwise most people would not score around 100 on the test. In putting together the questions for an IQ test, the testmakers are careful to select those items that can be answered by only 50 percent of the standardization group and to eliminate items that show different patterns of response. In addition, items are selected so that each question will more often be answered correctly by overall high scorers and will be least likely answered correctly by low scorers. Suppose, for instance, that John and Mary both were part of the standardization group and that John received a low overall score and Mary a high overall score. Any particular items that John answered correctly and that Mary did not answer correctly would then be eliminated from the test, since those items would be considered incapable of differentiating the intelligent person from the unintelligent person. In this way, low scorers are guaranteed against scoring higher, and high scorers are guaranteed against scoring lower.

Another manipulation of test items concerns male-female differences. There are certain tasks, such as tests of spatial-quantitative relations and mechanical tasks, on which males surpass females, and some tasks, such as memory and verbal ability, on which females surpass males. Intelligence test designers eliminated items that strongly favored either sex, and balanced remaining items so that both men and women have an equal chance of obtaining the same distribution of scores. On tests where that was too difficult to achieve, the designers eliminated sex differences by adjusting the conversion of raw scores into IQ scores by sex, thereby ensuring equity. Although it would also be possible to eliminate test items that account for differences in scores between ethnic groups, using the same procedures as were used in sex differences, the test designers have not done so, because these differences accord with their assumptions about intelligence.

There is a consensus among test designers as to what the various IQ scores indicate about the level or your intelligence, as follows:

IQ Score	Supposed Intelligence Level
130 +	Very superior
120–129	Superior
110–119	High average or Bright normal
90–109	Average
80– 89	Below average or Dull normal
70– 79	Borderline
69 and below	Mentally deficient or Mentally defective

Despite the fact that IQ tests are of dubious validity, they continue to play an important part in your life. So, as the old saying goes, "if you can't beat 'em, join 'em."

TIPS ON TAKING TESTS

Research has shown that coaching can help raise scores on standardized tests in two basic ways: by giving you some familiarity with the test-taking procedures and by giving you specific skills in handling the various questions you will be asked. The rest of this chapter is devoted to coaching you in these two areas.

Group Tests

As already mentioned, many publishing companies put out workbooks designed to help you take a variety of group tests, such as the SAT, GRE, and LSAT. These books are very helpful and you should by all means look them through before you take a test.

Workbooks give you sample tests that are like the actual test you will take, though obviously, they cannot provide you with copies of the exact test you will be taking. Many tests are published by the same companies that do the testing (SAT, GRE, Miller Analogies), and their tests are not available to the general public or to professionals. Some states, with truth-in-testing laws, do allow you to see the actual test taken, the correct answers, and a copy of your answer sheet after the fact, if you submit a written request and pay the specified fee. Some tests, however, like the Otis and Henmon-Nelson IQ tests, are sold to professionals who administer the tests. Although you cannot buy such a test yourself from the publisher, information about it is more readily available. Most examiners will not tell you beforehand what tests they will be giving you, although you should certainly ask, but you can check in the library and read whatever textbooks you can find on intelligence and whatever testing manuals you can find.

In addition to giving you a better idea of the specific types of questions each test covers, reading up on a test will also help you plan your test-taking strategy. Different tests are scored in different ways. Some just add up the number of correct answers to determine your score, and others penalize you for wrong answers. On the first type of test, it obviously pays to guess when you are not sure of an answer, but on the second type of test it may not pay. Workbooks and test manuals will help you know when you should and should not guess and even provide formulas for the degree of certainty you need to make guessing pay off. Workbooks and test manuals also acquaint you with time limits of the various tests and help you know how to apportion your time best. Some tests restrict the time for each section, whereas some set a time limit only for the whole test. In the latter situation, you can "borrow" time from the easier tasks to use on the more difficult ones. You will also be able to figure out how much time you can afford to spend on any one question.

When you take a large-scale standardized test at a testing center, you are usually required to bring along your own pencils —the instruction booklets distributed at the time you register for such tests will so inform you. When you take a test at a personnel department or at an individualized testing center, the pencils will usually be provided for you. Most tests are electronically scored, picking up impulses from your pencil marks. On such tests you will have to fill in a designated area with pencil shadings. Do not be compulsive about filling in the entire area because that wastes precious time. All you need to do is put in a fairly good sized blob. To speed up the filling-in process, bring along pencils that are not too sharp. If the point is already somewhat dulled, the shading process will go more quickly. If you make a wrong insertion, be careful to erase completely so there is no lead mark left for electronic scoring.

Individual Tests

To our knowledge, there are no workbooks on taking individual tests. Unlike the group tests, which are given on a mass basis at set intervals during the year and which change questions from test to test, the individual tests are always the same. Although you cannot buy a sample test unless you are a professional psychologist or psychometrician, you can learn a lot about individual tests from the test manuals, which are available in some libraries. These books will provide you with the questions contained on the verbal parts of the tests. Some people feel that it is cheating to know the questions beforehand. Because differences in cultural and socioeconomic backgrounds mean that people who take tests have had different amounts of exposure to and experience with the type of material on the test, becoming familiar with the test questions through a test manual is really no more cheating than is going to a prep school that trains you how to do well on the types of materials covered by IQ tests.

Unlike group tests, which are scored by machine, individual tests are scored by the examiner and some questions, particularly the verbal ones, can be scored for one or two credits. If an answer is not complete according to the scoring criteria, the examiner is supposed to ask you to explain more fully and give you the opportunity to raise your score. Be compliant, even if you think your answer is sufficient, and give as detailed an answer as you can. Most of the verbal test questions are untimed, but some, like arithmetic, may be timed, even though the examiner might not tell you this. If you see a stopwatch or a wristwatch being used, you know that you are being timed; answer as quickly as possible so as not to lose points. Most often, the so-called performance problems, like jigsaw puzzles and coding, are timed, so work as fast as you can, even if you are not warned to do so by the examiner.

When individual IQ tests are used, the examiner often presents the IQ score along with a written summary about you. The examiner's overall impressions about you—how you look, how you respond to questions, how you interact with the examiner— will very likely influence the way the summary is written. The examiner may decide that your scores represent your upper limit, or that your scores indicate a potential for higher functioning, depending on the impression you have made. So look alert and be cooperative.

THE IMPORTANCE
OF VALUES IN SCORES

Testmakers have very definite, although erroneous, notions about the nature of intelligence. Their attitudes about what it is and who has it influence the way tests are constructed and IQs determined. The values of the testmakers also influence the way your responses are scored. Some questions, particularly those that test your comprehension, are based on value judgments and therefore have no absolute right or wrong answers. If you want to get a high IQ score, you must give responses that are in accord with the testmaker's values, even if they are not your own. Basically, IQ tests credit answers that demonstrate respect for authority and acceptance of established values and do not credit responses that demonstrate independence of thought and rejection of popular morality.

The Wechsler Intelligence Scale for Adults, for example, asks, in its comprehension subtest, "What is the thing to do if you are the first person at the movies to see smoke and fire?" The only full-credit response for this question involves reporting the problem to "a person in authority on the scene": "Report it to the manager or the usher." If you respond in a way that demonstrates readiness for direct action and independence, you may fail the item; according to the scoring manual, "Go for water" gets no credit and "Get a fire extinguisher" is not included as a scorable response. You can only get credit for trying to put the fire out if there is "recognition that responsible action" is "not so immediately effective" as referring the problem to an authority. Thus, you can get half-credit for the response "try to put the fire out or call the fire department," but no credit if you just try to put the fire out by yourself. The test assumes that the fire can be handled more competently by others and that you should not interfere with established procedures, even if it takes longer for you to find the manager than it does to find the extinguisher or if you should happen to be a trained firefighter. On this question, the test is more concerned with conformity than intelligent behavior and actually gives credit for nonintelligent behavior!

Another question on this test asks why one should keep away from "bad company." The question assumes that everyone agrees on what constitutes bad company. We happen to think that bad company is boring company, but if we answered that you should stay away from bad company because it is not intellectually fulfilling, we would not get any credit. If you accept the test-maker's implied definition of bad company as persons who are immoral, then you are also expected to go along with the premise that you should keep away from such people. As you might expect, full credit on this question requires a response that you will be corrupted or improperly influenced by bad company. The testmaker's view does not include the possibility that you might be strong enough to withstand the influence of bad company or possibly influence bad company to become good.

Values also crop up in nonverbal questions. The Stanford-Binet, for example, asks two questions in which the test-taker must select the prettier looking person. The correct woman, according to the test, is the Anglo-Saxon stereotype. The same criterion is used to determine the better-looking man. Children who identify with the face that does not live up to the aesthetic ideal of our culture lose credits. The fact that children in different ethnic and racial groups might have different conceptions of beauty does not seem to have occurred to the testmakers.

Stereotyped aesthetic notions show up on other tests as well. On the Pintner-Cunningham Primary Test, children are asked to select the nicest house of three. The houses vary in terms of door and window placement. The house that offers completely symmetrical placement of windows in a conventional pattern is scored as the correct response. The houses that show variation in placement from the standard pattern are considered incorrect because they are different. We happen to find one of the wrong answers more aesthetically pleasing. The placement of the windows on different levels not only enlivens the façade but suggests a more interesting multileveled interior as well. When you're taking an IQ test, put out of your mind momentarily everything written in this book about creativity and negative thinking. Improve your score by providing conventional answers to all questions that incorporate value judgments.

TYPICAL QUESTIONS

The questions on IQ tests are chosen to tap as wide a range as possible of the mental functions that are presumed to make up intelligence. Another consideration is a practical one, that they lend themselves to a test format. A large part of most IQ tests is taken up with verbal questions, because it is generally agreed that verbal skills are a very important aspect of intelligence and because verbal skills are easy to measure. Verbal questions consist of straight vocabulary items, or word definition questions, as well as many other types of questions that depend on your vocabulary: verbal analogies, antonyms (opposites), verbal classifications, and reading comprehension.

With the recognition that vocabulary-building is important to test-taking, many good workbooks on building vocabulary skills have become available. Practically every preparatory book for the SAT and its variants contains a special vocabulary section with a basic word list you should know, definitions of those words, and tips on building up your vocabulary, including lists of prefixes and common word roots. Also available are such preparatory books as *1100 Words You Need to Know*, among others. Because vocabulary enlargement is a fundamental tool in information-processing as well as in test-taking, we recommend that if your vocabulary is limited, you get one of these books. If working on vocabulary-building sounds like drudgery to you, try making it into a family game for the breakfast or dinner table, or practice vocabulary-building with a friend as you bike or jog, or write a letter to an imaginary friend using all the new words you have learned in any given day in one paragraph. Once you get started on vocabulary-building, you will probably find it fascinating and fun rather than a chore. The vocabulary workbooks provide interesting insights into the language—how the words were derived, the borrowing from different language groups, the various prefixes and roots and their meanings, and so on. Time spent in studying word origins helps build your vocabulary by making it possible for you to understand new words once you can analyze them into their component parts and roots.

Vocabulary Questions

On a paper-and-pencil test, a vocabulary question will usually be in the form of a multiple choice.

Example _____

Choose the word which is most similar in meaning to the underlined word:

parity: (1) miniature (2) score (3) similarity (4) alottment (5) event

On these questions there are often words among the alternatives that you might be apt to choose if you are unsure of the correct meaning. In the example above, people unfamiliar with *parity* might be misled into checking *score* because of the relationship between *score* and *par,* rather than *similarity.*

Vocabulary questions on individual tests require you to give the examiner your own definition:

Example _____

What does emerald mean?

When answering these open-ended questions, it is always a good idea to give a detailed response, since the credit given for your answer depends on its fullness. The examiner is usually instructed to ask you to expand on your response if it does not rate full credit by saying something like "Tell me more about it" or "Would you please explain that further?" Don't worry about how much time you take answering; vocabulary items are not scored for time. It might help to keep the following criteria in mind when defining a word; they are taken from the two-point (full credit) list of criteria on the Wechsler Intelligence Scales:

- a synonym
- a major use
- one or more major features, or many minor features
- category in which the word belongs
- for verbs, an example of action

Vocabulary questions are frequently asked in the form of antonyms. Instead of having to select a word similar in meaning to the test word, you are asked to select a word opposite in meaning.

Example _____

Choose the word that means the opposite of the underlined word:

adamant: (1) flexible (2) original (3) official (4) persistent (5) arrogant

On antonym questions the testmakers usually include a word that is similar in meaning to the underlined word as well as a word that is a correct antonym. In the example above, a nervous test subject might be apt to select *persistent* as the answer since the two words are close in meaning, rather than the correct response, *flexible*, which is opposite in meaning to *adamant*. The testmakers purposely try to catch you up, since their concept of intelligence includes ability to follow instructions.

Verbal Analogies

The purpose of verbal analogies is to test your ability to reason as well as the breadth of your vocabulary. Analogy questions on some tests, therefore, deal with relatively simple words, but higher level tests will include more obscure words. Many years ago, when we took the Miller Analogies Test, one of the words on the test was *marsupial*—not that difficult if you know your biology, but not your everyday conversational word.

Verbal analogy questions appear in various forms, depending on the test. Some are written out in words:

square is to cube as _____ is to _____
(1) irregular to symmetrical
(2) area to perimeter
(3) circle to sphere
(4) parallelogram to trapezoid
(5) obtuse to acute

Other verbal analogies are written out in symbols:

square : cube : :
(1) irregular : symmetrical
(2) area : perimeter

(3) circle : sphere
(4) parallelogram : trapezoid
(5) obtuse : acute

To answer this question correctly, you have to figure out the relationship between the question words, in this instance, square and cube. A square is two-dimensional and a cube is a three-dimensional figure that looks like a square when projected on a flat surface. The same relationship holds between a circle and a sphere, so (3) is the correct answer.

Intelligence tests usually focus on particular types of relationships, as described in the list below:

A broad category is compared to a member of that category:
human : boy = vehicle : automobile

A whole to one of its parts:
body : arm = car : wheel

A cause to its effect:
rain : flood = sun : drought

A greater degree to a lesser degree:
jubilant : happy = freezing : cool

An instrument to its function:
scale : measurement = car : transportation

A positive to a negative:
honesty : dishonesty = bravery : cowardice

A person to a characteristic:
adult : maturity = child : dependence

A person to a tool:
tailor : needle = artist : brush

A person to a profession:
teacher : education = author : literature

Similarities

Similarities questions usually appear on individual IQ tests. You are asked to describe how two things are similar. The pairs in these questions may be objects, like an apple and a peach, or concepts, like good and bad. In scoring your answers, the examiner is looking for not just a correct answer, but for an answer expressing the highest level of generalization; that is usually the category or class to which things belong. The full credit answer to how an apple and peach are the same would be that "they are both fruits." Other answers, such as "they are both good to eat," or "they both grow on trees," are correct, but only are scored for partial credit, because they deal in concrete characteristics rather than an abstract category.

Sometimes the scoring criteria are more flexible. For instance, on the Wechsler Intelligence Scale for Children (revised form), the question as to how scissors and copper pan are similar is scored for full credit if you say they are both made of metal, as well as if you say they are both household utensils. In this instance, full credit is given for recognizing shared characteristics as well as general category.

Similarities questions are tests of your conceptual thinking. You might find it helpful to refer back to the chapter "Modes of Thinking," which explains the differences among concept grouping principles. When taking a similarities test, if you are not sure of your answer, try to give more than one response.

Interpretation of Proverbs

These questions present you with a well-known proverb and ask that you provide the meaning. On a group test, you will be offered a multiple-choice selection and on an individual test you will be asked to supply your own answer. A typical question would be, "What is the meaning of the saying 'Still waters run deep'?" In answering these questions, you should supply a general meaning such as "Quiet people may be very profound thinkers," rather than a specific one such as "A river that is deep does not have much surface movement." Again, answer with the broadest generalization you can think of.

Sentence Completion

Answering these questions depends on your vocabulary. You are required to fill in the missing word or pair of words in a sentence. Usually the missing words will be rather difficult, because you are expected to use the context of the sentence to figure out what the words mean. The word you choose must, of course, make sense when inserted into the sentence. An example follows:

> Many people believe that the _____ of IQ scores and race is based on a _____ relationship between the two.

> Choose the correct words to complete the sentence:
> (a) correlation–causal
> (b) magnitude–definitive
> (c) inequality–biased
>
> Correct answer: (a)

Reading Comprehension

On these questions you have to read a selected passage and then answer a series of questions. Because reading-comprehension questions are timed, it is important that you read well—for speed and comprehension. Check the section on reading in the chapter "Processing Verbal Information" if you think you do not read as well as you could.

Following Instructions

These questions ask you to follow a set of directions, usually somewhat complicated, as follows:

> If the difference between eleven and six is more than five, make a cross in the first box.

> ☐☐☐☐☐☐

Sometimes the directions will require you to compare figures instead of numbers. Take the following question, for instance:

> If the vertical line is longer than the horizontal line put a P in the parentheses but if this is not the case put a Q next to the longer figure.
>
> ( ) _____

Math Questions

Most intelligence tests have a variety of questions requiring math skills. The Wechsler scales have a subtest limited to basic arithmetic, but the group placement tests, such as the SAT, have an extensive math section requiring knowledge of algebra and geometry. If your math is shaky and you want to do well on the placement tests, you had best get a math review book. Some typical questions are described below.

Number series completion

This type of question shows up fairly often and, in fact, makes up roughly 5 percent of the Otis test. Example: What number should come next: 3 5 6 8 9 11 ___? To answer this question, you have to figure out the pattern of the differences between the numbers, in this example it is plus two, plus one, plus two, plus one, with the correct answer being 12.

Math analogies

These questions, like verbal analogies, require that you determine the relationship between a pair of numbers and replicate that pattern in the answer. For example: $1/6 : 2/12 = 1/4 :$ _____ Since the numbers in the sample set are in the same proportion but doubled, the correct answer is 2/8.

Percent Problems

Problems involving the calculation of percentages are quite popular and are presented in word problems. You need to know both how to figure out a given percent of any number and how to calculate the original number of which a given number represents a certain percentage. For example: If you get a 10 percent discount on a fifteen-dollar item, how much do you have to pay? Another example: Thirty is 10 percent of what number?

Days Worked

This problem format seems to be a favorite of test constructors. Example: "If six men can finish a job in three days, how many men will be needed to finish it in one day?"

Word Problems

In addition to the fairly simple addition/subtraction, multiplication/division, and percentage problems presented as word problems, intelligence tests sometimes also include word problems dealing with rate of speed and distance covered, rate of work and time needed, and conversion from one measure to another (inches to feet). It is a good idea to familiarize yourself with these types of problems before taking a test if they give you difficulty.

Memory Questions

Some of the individual tests include memory questions. Most frequently these are Digit Span, in which you are required to repeat back a series of numbers. The series go as high as nine digits. Sometimes you are required to repeat the digits backwards. Another memory test consists of repeating back a sentence. It is important that you repeat the sentence back exactly. The examiner is not interested in how well you get the gist of the sentence, but in your ability to replicate it.

Figural Classification

These questions ask you to select the figure that is different from the others. For example, "Select the figure which is different from the other four:"

B K g P V

Here the answer is obviously g because it is lower case, while the others are upper case. Figures may vary along other dimensions, of course. In addition to size, a figure may not belong in a series because of curvedness or angularity, openness or closedness, having overlapping parts, orientation in space, shading, and so on.

Figural Reasoning

These problems are somewhat similar to number series in that you must discern the relationship in a series of figures and then choose the correct figure to complete the pattern. Look at the following example:

@   *   (

@@   **   ((

@@   **   ?

Choose the Correct Answer:

((   ))   ⌒   ≍

In this problem the figures change from column to column and from row to row. In the first row there is one figure, in the second row there are two figures, and in the third row there are two figures turned upside down. This last change is obscured by the fact that the asterisk, when turned upside down, looks the same as right-side up. These types of problems can become quite difficult. Figures can be presented with changes in shape, shading, size, number, position (movement in a plane or flipover of a figure), superimposition of figures, and unique additions of figures (in which only similar parts of figures are retained). The various changes can become so complex that someone has written a book devoted almost solely to how to take tests of this type. In case you want to perfect this skill, look at *Up the IQ* by Paul Jacobs.

Block Design

This is part of the Wechsler Intelligence Scales. The subject is given a set of blocks up to nine in number, each with different-colored sides, and presented with various designs to copy using the blocks. Each design has to be completed within a time limit, with extra points given for speed. Some toy shops sell versions of this test, along with sample designs for you to complete, and they are good practice for taking the test.

Picture Arrangement

On this test you are presented with a series of pictures, which must be arranged in the proper sequence so that they tell a sensible story. Many of the sequences are cartoon series. You can practice this test by having a friend cut up the Sunday funnies and give them to you in shuffled order. A sequence of five to six cartoon frames without words is about the right length.

Picture Completion

The test-taker is presented with pictures that have missing parts, which must be identified. The missing parts include such items as a nose, threads on the base of a light bulb, the shadow of a house, and so forth.

Jigsaw Puzzles

These come in many different forms from the simple, on children's tests, to the complex, on the Wechsler Adult Intelligence Scale. The puzzles can be difficult because they are presented without identifying features such as color or surface designs. Also, you are not told what to construct. These puzzles are timed, and extra credit is given for speedy construction.

Coding

On coding tests you are required to write in the correct symbols for a series of numbers, following a code that is provided. For example:

1	2	3	4	5	6	7	8	9
)	+	$	%	!	&	=	*	"

Now fill in the correct symbol under each digit:

9 5 1 3 7 2 6 4 8 5 9 7 3 1 9 etc.

– – – – – – – – – – – – – – –

This test is timed, with extra points for speedy completion. The faster you learn the symbols so you don't have to keep referring back to the sample, the better. To practice for this test it is quite simple to prepare your own practice sheets using home-devised codes such as the one above. The symbols may vary from test to test, but once you get in the swing of it, you can do it well on any test.

THE INTELLIGENCE POTENTIAL

In recent years there has been more and more recognition that the IQ tests do not measure intelligence, but rather, the level of intellectual development that has been achieved. To get closer to understanding a person's intellectual potential, it is argued that we do not need to know what a person has already learned, but what that person's capacity for learning is. With this view in mind, one of the recent trends in test development has been in the measurement of learning potential. This trend has taken hold most notably in Israel, under the direction of Reuven Feuerstein, and in the Soviet Union.

Feuerstein and his colleagues have developed a tool called the Learning Potential Assessment Device. During the testing session, which lasts between four to five hours, the examiner tests to see how far a child can go with a task when the examiner intervenes with helpful instructions along the way. Children who test at a retarded level on standard tests often show the capacity for high-level intellectual performance with the benefit of such mediated experience. Feuerstein's test-teach-test method allows the examiner to follow the flow of a child's thinking processes, to diagnose problem areas, and to give the child necessary thinking tools that have been lacking in the child's environment.

Testing in the Soviet Union also distinguishes between a child's actual and potential level of development. The actual level is viewed as the performance on a standardized test and the potential level as the performance that can be achieved with assistance in the course of testing. The difference is referred to as the *zone of potential development.* It is assumed that children with a wide zone have greater cognitive potential, although they may be learning-disabled, and that children with a narrow zone are those who have limited potential and are, perhaps, brain-damaged.

The concept of intelligence potential is a step forward. It recognizes a major problem inherent in IQ testing and correctly interprets IQ test results as a measure of current performance, not of fixed performance. Even so, the concept takes a rather limited view in that it assumes that potential is fixed. We believe that it is as difficult to measure potential accurately as it is to measure intelligence accurately. Once an individual starts using untapped mental abilities, it is possible that more potentialities will emerge than currently meet the eye. Further, the concept focuses on verbal skills and left-brain functions rather than on the full panoply of human abilities, again giving a one-sided view of human potential and a one-sided emphasis to its development.

EMOTIONS AND INTELLIGENCE

We tend to see our emotions and intelligence as separate and incompatible parts of ourselves. To stay clearheaded, we are told, we must keep our emotions out. Certainly it is true that strong emotions can interfere with one's thinking as, for example, when you are too excited to think, too angry to be fair, or too preoccupied with worry to react to some obvious event right in front of your nose. But that view of our emotions is much too limited and ignores their positive contribution.

Emotions help as well as hinder intelligence. They are an integral part of intellectual functioning, rather than separate from or fundamentally antagonistic to intelligence. In fact, without emotions we would have no intelligence. One of the reasons we ignore the positive role of emotions is, paradoxically, because it is so basic to our being. We tend to take the things we depend on for granted, noticing their absence rather than their presence. Ordinarily we are not aware of being in good health, although we are very conscious of our ill health. With emotions, too, we tend to be oblivious of how they work *for* us, becoming concerned only when they get in the way.

Another reason the positive contribution of emotions is dismissed is because of the emphasis in Western civilization on so-called objective thought. In the pursuit of science, people have come to overvalue what is called pure thought and cold logic and to denigrate emotions as a polluting influence rather than accept them as a necessary and positive force. This chapter explores how emotions can work for you as well as against you, so that you can make the most intelligent use of your feelings.

THE BASIC MODE OF KNOWING

Emotions in themselves are carriers of intelligence. Like thoughts, emotions stem from our brains, but from the evolutionarily older midbrain rather than from the more recently developed cortex. Emotions and thoughts are both part of our repertoire of responses for dealing with the world. While emotions are distinct from thought and logic, they are not of a lower order. They serve us differently, but are just as important in intelligent behavior.

If people are transplanted from one culture to another where they cannot understand the language and what is being spoken, they still have no difficulty understanding the emotions being expressed by the speakers. Even in the absence of visual cues, research has shown that people can identify the emotions expressed in recordings when the content has been made unintelligible by electronic masking. Our emotional impressions are immediate and strong, preceding thought. As the old saying recognizes, the heart knows before the head. In earlier times emotional impressions were considered to be a valid source of information. Indeed, the revealing power of emotions is recognized even in the Bible, which equates love with *knowing*.

When our emotions are aroused, they serve to mobilize us to action. If we are threatened, we react with anger that helps to maintain our physical safety or psychic integrity. If we are welcomed, we feel love to draw us close to those who enhance our spiritual well-being. Emotional responses are organized primarily in that part of the midbrain known as the limbic system. Within the limbic system is the hypothalamus, which influences the internal state of our bodies. As our emotions undergo shifts, our breathing rate, heart rate, and other body functions change so that our total activity level is adjusted to meet the needs of the situation. In this manner emotions are the basic survival mechanism of all animals, more refined in humans, and available for intelligent response.

THE MOTIVE POWER BEHIND INTELLIGENCE

Emotions not only provide their own intelligence, but they are basic to all forms of intellectual endeavor. A fundamental requirement of an active intelligence is motivation, and it is the emotions that fuel the exploratory drive that engages our intellect with the environment. Without that drive, we would not exercise our intelligence.

Because emotions tend to be seen as a negative factor that interferes with reason, the important motive power of emotions has been largely ignored in theories of intelligence. Recognizing the role that emotions play in intelligence, Ward C. Halstead, a Chicago psychologist, postulated a *power factor*, which he believed was necessary to motivate the mind to explore and concentrate.

Virtually all great achievements of the mind come about through an intense engagement with some intellectual problem. The emotions provide the driving power and satisfaction that pushes the mind to attain its exceptional accomplishments. The same principle applies, of course, to other areas of achievement. The skills of an artist or athlete are developed through a strong emotional drive for mastery. Without that motivation, the persistent application required to develop those skills is not possible. To succeed at anything, including raising intelligence, requires motivated effort. Thomas Edison recognized the importance of this principle in commenting that "Invention is 10 percent inspiration and 90 percent perspiration."

It has been estimated that we have fifty-odd emotions. Some, like anger and fear, are more primitive; others, such as hope and guilt are more complex and involve the cortex as well as the midbrain. Without these emotions, we would not be able to sustain the right mood for our assorted endeavors. The various emotions differ in the way they interact with intelligence. Some feelings, particularly self-confidence, joy, and trust, are conducive to intelligent behavior, but many others have a problematical role. We will discuss the more helpful emotions first.

THE HELPFUL EMOTIONS

Self-Confidence

People who are confident about their ability make demands on their intelligence. People who are not give up too soon and fail to challenge their minds. Your confidence in your abilities has a crucial effect on how much of your intellectual potential is developed.

As you grow up, what you expect of yourself is a reflection of what others, mostly your parents and teachers, expect of you. Studies conducted by David McClelland at Harvard on the achievement motive found that children achieve at above average levels when their parents expect them to do well and to behave independently. These children absorb and then actualize a *can-*

do attitude. Teachers also play an important role in shaping performance. In a well-known study, teachers were told that certain children would show unusual academic development during the year. Although these children were no different from others in the class, the children so labeled actually did better than their classmates on a group intelligence test at the end of the year. Their teachers' expectations that they would succeed actually helped them to perform at a higher level. The expectations of society also shape the child's performance, and these expectations are usually too low. The normal school system underestimates children's ability to learn and thereby diminishes their sense of competence. The fact that many Soviet high school students can do calculus and speak English does not mean that they are smarter than American students, but that it is not difficult to learn those skills when it is taken for granted that one can do so. Too many American students expect, instead, that they have a math block or that they can't learn a foreign language. This undermines their confidence to learn and helps create math blocks and the inability to speak foreign languages.

If you look at the biographies of exceptional people, you will find that most had parents who helped to give them confidence in their abilities. Their parents not only encouraged their endeavors, but expressed a great deal of admiration for their accomplishments. A recent study by *Family Circle* on fifty prominent Americans revealed that, from early childhood on, their mothers set up expectations of their success and confidence in their ability to attain it. Along with emphasis on learning and participation in adult activities went encouragement, reward, and an expressed confidence in the child's capability. Studies that have focused on the personality characteristics of the creative adult similarly find a marked degree of self-confidence in such persons. All the available evidence shows that a genuine belief in your own capacity to be more intelligent is a fundamental prerequisite to realizing your possibilities.

Although we are born with vast potentials, most of us lose confidence in our intellectual worth as we grow up. Few parents realize that intelligence must be nurtured and leave their children's intellectual development in the hands of the schools. Because of their lack of time or patience, many parents actually inhibit their children's intellectual growth by chiding them for asking too many questions, butting in on adult conversations, and the like. Thus, intellectual curiosity may lead to punishment rather than reward, inhibiting the child's drive to learn and threatening the child's self-assurance. When children enter school, self-confidence in their intellectual worth is often further eroded. Teachers are prone to categorize children according to their assumed intellectual capacity and thereby set levels of expectations that are too low. The children, in turn, grow up thinking too little of themselves and not expecting very much of themselves. With these feelings it is impossible to make full use of one's intelligence and the first job is to restore confidence in one's abilities.

Exercise

Positive Self-Evaluation

Most people underrate their abilities or do not recognize them at all. If you were asked to name your ten greatest accomplishments you probably would hem and haw and then say you haven't really accomplished anything very much. This is just not so. You have accomplished a great deal but don't give yourself credit for it. Let's prove the point. Get paper and pencil and start making a list of all the things you do well. If you are having trouble thinking of things, start reviewing every area of your life—not just work or school. What about hobbies, sports, personal relationships, community activities? Write down everything that comes to mind that you do well, even if at first thought it seems unimportant. When you have twenty items on your list you can stop. Read over them carefully and check the ten that you are proudest of. Now you can analyze those activities to see what they entail. Here is an example:

Your Ten Most Important Accomplishments	Mechanical Aptitude	Planning Ahead	Perceptual Acuity	Problem-Solving Ability	Creative Ability	Organizational Ability	Decision-Making Ability
cooking well	x	x			x	x	
good golf game	x	x	x	x			
effective on PTA committee		x		x		x	x
driving well	x		x	x			x
balancing checkbook		x		x		x	
crossword puzzles			x	x	x		
sewing clothes	x		x		x		
guitar-playing	x		x		x		
speak second language			x	x			
can help friends when troubled		x		x		x	x

Each activity that you do well requires special intellectual talents and abilities. You may think your ability to cook well is unimportant, but it involves mechanical aptitude (cutting the onions, flipping the pancakes so they don't break); planning ahead (don't forget to buy the string beans, if you don't chill the dough for at least two hours before it won't be flaky); creative ability (I think I'll substitute chocolate chips for the grated orange rind; if I use the pineapple husk as a serving dish, it should look attractive); organizational ability (there are only four burners but six dishes, so if I cook the potatoes in the bottom of the double boiler, the peas can steam on top at the same time). Your cooking skills, like your ability to drive a car, organize a committee meeting, and balance personal finances require the same varied aspects of intelligence as deriving a mathematical formula, locating viruses under a microscope, or heading a large business. One tends to dismiss those skills because they are not embodied in a prestigious or high-paying occupation, but they require the same fundamental capacities: mechanical aptitude, perceptual acuity, planning ability, decision-making ability, creative ability, organizational ability, and more. When you give yourself credit for what you can do, and expect more of yourself, you will give your intelligence room to grow.

Joy and Trust

Other feelings that enhance intelligence are joy and trust. Although these feelings are, of course, beneficial in many ways, their particular value to intelligence is that they encourage us to be open to new experiences.

When you are feeling joyous, it is usually accompanied by feelings of confidence and optimism about your possibilities. The feeling of joy lets you exercise your intelligence because it encourages you to try new things, take risks, and expand yourself. When you experience joy, you are open to life, and the more open you are the more can come in. People's bursts of creativity often occur during their joyful moments when they are most willing to explore and try their wings.

The benefits of trust are similar. When we are able to trust, we can allow ourselves to experiment with new perspectives and new experiences. Lack of trust closes us off defensively. Trust comes from faith in others, but even more from confidence in our own ability to deal with the situations we meet.

Joy, trust, and self-confidence have a mutually reinforcing effect on each other and on intelligence. The more you can bring them into your life, the more intelligent you will become. And the more intelligent you become, the more you will guide yourself into experiences that allow those beneficial emotions to flourish.

HOW EMOTIONS CAN LIMIT INTELLIGENCE

So far we have been talking about the positive effects of emotion on intelligence. Emotions can also have a limiting effect on intelligence, but it is not so much their existence as it is our inability to integrate them constructively in our behavior that creates problems. When we are confronted with feelings that are too unpleasant, or too threatening to our sense of security, we set up defenses against them to maintain our equilibrium. These defenses, which include denying what we feel, distorting what we see, or rationalizing what we think, act as shock absorbers and temporary morale-boosters, but the price we pay is a blunting of our intelligence. As we regulate our awareness to levels that are manageable for our adjustment, we also shut ourselves off from important data about the world. The following are five main tricks our mind can play on us to make us feel better.

Selective Inattention

This technique lets us avoid seeing what we cannot handle emotionally. A person who is envious of a rival may, for example, ignore the latter's good points, only seeing the negatives. In contrast, a mother who is overly involved in her child may be blind to her youngster's shortcomings, seeing only praiseworthy qualities. The member of the audience who is out to impress the gathering with his questions may not attend to the fact that everyone is yawning. The ardent suitor may not be registering the fact that his sweetheart keeps removing his hand. And so it goes—emotional needs can make you overlook whole areas of importance. Selective inattention may keep you from feeling bad momentarily, but it interferes with clear thinking and reaching accurate conclusions.

Distortion

Feelings not only block perception; they can also get in the way of accurate perception. That is the main reason why different observers at the scene of an accident or a crime often give different versions of what has occurred. The bystander who feels guilty that he did not intervene may describe the assailant as much bigger than he actually was. The bigot may describe the assailant as dark-skinned rather than as a white person seen in the shadows. Firsthand accounts can be notoriously discrepant with one another. Distortions apply to self-perceptions as well. A modest person may see his or her accomplishments as minimal, while an immodest person may see the same sort of accomplishment as a major feat.

In the chapter "Enhancing Perception," we described how children from low socioeconomic backgrounds saw the size of coins as larger than they were and how adults distorted their perceptions of the size of rods to conform to those of others because of a need for acceptance. The tendency to distort occurs at all ages and among all kinds of people, varying with the strength of one's emotional needs on one hand and ability to deal with them on the other. People who are aware of how easily one can be swayed tend to be more accurate in their perceptions.

Making Exceptions

Sometimes it is not possible to distort reality that is emotionally disturbing. When that happens, another line of defense is to shrug off the upsetting information as unimportant or atypical. "That's just a fluke"; "It couldn't happen again in a million years." To justify the rejection of information that does not fit one's needs, the familiar adage that "the exception proves the rule" is invoked. The way this phrase is interpreted is itself an emotionally based distortion. The intended meaning is that the exception tests the validity of the rule: if the rule cannot accommodate the exception, the rule is wrong. Popular use of the phrase twists it to mean that the exceptional case that does not conform to the rule proves the rule is right!

Reinterpreting

Just in case selective inattention, distortion, and making exceptions do not suffice in dealing with emotionally unpleasant material, there is still another device available: reinterpretation. We can call a rival aggressive and cutthroat, while our own similar behavior is seen instead as putting our best foot forward and getting ahead. We may interpret the noisy behavior of other people's children as ill-mannered and reinterpret this behavior when displayed by our own children as creative expression. We may see the physical advances of an attractive person as sexy but interpret similar advances from an unattractive person as lascivious. We may interpret our questions about a neighbor as friendly curiosity but interpret another's questions as nosiness. Reinterpretation allows us to avoid, at least temporarily, acknowledging disturbing feelings, but by the same token it limits our ability for intelligent assessment.

Denying

The most flagrant defense against unpleasant feelings is to deny outright the information that sets them off. We have all heard people declare, "It can't be true," or "You don't mean it" when facing accidents, deaths, or other sudden traumatic experiences. To give us time to get used to the painful feelings evoked by such situations, we try to defend ourselves by an initial period of disbelief. Usually after a while we can face the truth. However, when denial becomes a characteristic way of dealing with threatening emotions, this defense becomes a very serious limitation of our intelligence because it forces us to narrow drastically our knowledge of the world as it is. Unless you confront the feelings that are causing the denial, you will be severely hampering your capacity to function in an intelligent way.

To reiterate, the less we are able to tolerate our feelings, the more we narrow our intelligence to reduce their disturbing impact. The more we are able to tolerate our feelings, the more intelligent use we can make of them. No one can be completely without emotional defenses, but by being alert to them, we can lessen their restricting effect on our intellectual processes. Look now at some of the problematic emotions and see how we can deal with them without sacrificing intellectual integrity.

THE DISTURBING EMOTIONS

Anger

Angry feelings are aroused when we feel we are being used, deprived, or treated unfairly. The value of anger is that it gets us to react to situations that represent a threat to us. If we did not feel angry when misused, we would tend to sit back and passively accept whatever life dealt out to us.

The problem with anger is that it can easily escalate and cause an overreaction. We recognize the loss of intelligence that results in such situations when we say that a person is blind with rage, or blows his top. These reactions obviously keep one from addressing the problem at hand intelligently.

Often, when we become very angry it is because the anger-inducing situation triggers other disturbing emotions as well. When others mistreat us, it can arouse dormant feelings of unworthiness and fear about our ability to cope with the threat. If you can separate the various feelings fueling your anger, it will enable you to respond more intelligently.

Anxiety

Your anxiety and intelligence have a complicated love-hate relationship with each other. Contrary to popular belief, anxiety is not necessarily bad for you. Very high and very low levels of anxiety are generally counterproductive to intelligent behavior, but a modicum of anxiety can be very useful where your intelligence is concerned.

When you feel anxious, your body undergoes subtle changes that make you more alert and keep you activated. Your adrenalin flows, your heart beats faster, your pulse rate increases. If anxiety becomes too great, you tend to become distracted by these bodily changes and to focus inward, losing your perspective of what is going on. In the absence of any anxiety, your whole system is inclined to be phlegmatic. With optimal anxiety, you are tuned up to react quickly and keenly.

Experiments have shown that anxiety has an important influence on learning. In one study, learning ability was examined under three levels of anxiety—very low, moderate, and high— that were created by the degree of importance attached to the learning. The "moderate anxiety" group learned best. The "very low anxiety" group lacked the motivation to learn well, and the "very high anxiety" group stuck to obvious responses, being too tense to experiment with better solutions.

In addition to its direct interference with intelligent behavior, high anxiety also affects intelligence indirectly. People who are very anxious sense that their anxiety impedes their performance. This makes them lose self-confidence and become dependent on the thinking of others. This dependence makes them intellectually less active and undermines their self-confidence still further.

If you tend to be anxious and tense most of the time, when you get into an anxiety-provoking situation your anxiety is likely to increase to the point where it interferes with your intelligent behavior. To prevent this from happening you need to learn how to reduce excessive anxiety.

Exercise

You will be able to use your intelligence more fully by learning to relax. Basically, all relaxation procedures involve putting yourself in a comfortable position, regulating your breathing, and doing visualization exercises that help to reduce muscle tension, as described in the steps listed below.

1. Pick a quiet place, free from disturbances, with fresh air circulating.

2. Place yourself in a comfortable position, either sitting or prone. If you sit, do so in a straight-backed chair, sitting upright, legs uncrossed and both feet on the floor, hands on your lap. If prone, lie on a smooth, firm surface with arms at your sides.

3. Loosen your tie, belt, shoelaces or any other tight clothing.

4. Breathe regularly and mentally check over your body for tension spots, starting with the scalp of your head and moving downwards towards your toes. Particularly check for the common tension spots such as stiffness of jaw, tenseness between shoulder blades or in the small of the back, clenching of fists, tightness of toes, or whatever your particular tension points are. As you focus on each tension area, loosen it up.

5. Slow down the rhythm of your breathing by focusing on your inhalations and exhalations, and saying, subvocally, the word *Relax* every time you exhale. Continue to slow down your breathing rate by counting slowly to six for each inhalation and exhalation. When you feel comfortable with this rate, try increasing the count to seven and then to eight, but only if it does not create discomfort for you.

6. Now visualize the air you are breathing as a cool refreshing breeze that flows through your body and carries away all tension with it. Again focus on each area of your body; start with your head and work your way down. See the breeze relaxing your scalp, your face, your jaw, and so on down your body. As you inhale, visualize the air flowing in, and as you exhale see all the tensions being expelled with your breath. When your whole body is relaxed, visualize the air flowing through it without any resistance.

7. Get up slowly, do a few stretches, and then go about your business.

Another excellent way to relax is to learn meditation techniques. In addition to lowering anxiety, meditation, by altering your mind's point of focus, filters out disturbing emotions and helps tune you in to the inner sources of intelligence. Meditation techniques are described in the next chapter, "Hidden Powers of the Mind."

Envy

Compared to other troubling emotions, envy has virtually nothing to commend it. Envy results from feeling deprived, not necessarily because we don't have enough but because someone else has more. We may, for example, be contentedly driving down the road in our Chevrolet enjoying the scenery, and suddenly feel a surge of envy as we are passed by a jet-set couple in an open Mercedes-Benz. Envy can be experienced regardless of how much one has attained. A corporate president, no matter how successful and highly paid, might envy a competitor for having a fancier office or still higher income. The basis of envy is the false sense of competition we feel with people who we do not necessarily even know. Their possession of some quantity or quality that we do not have makes us seem lowered in our own eyes. Envy distorts reality by preventing us from evaluating our situations realistically and propels us to imitative rather than to useful behavior.

People who are envious are described as being consumed with envy. They have little energy left for intelligent and constructive behavior because their resources are eaten up by the force of their resentment. Whereas anger helps us to turn our energy outwards, envy makes us turn in on ourselves.

To keep envy from compromising your intelligence, recognize it for what it is: a feeling of irrational deprivation that indicates dissatisfaction with yourself. Feeling resentful that you don't have what the other guy has makes it harder for you to focus on getting for yourself what you need.

Guilt

Guilt is usually considered to be a useless and constraining emotion. The vogue in pop psychology today is to tell you to stop feeling guilty. Despite its bad name, guilt is actually a helpful emotion and an intelligent response. It lets you know when you are not living up to some standard of behavior that is important to you. For example, we feel guilt when we avoid intelligent behavior or in other ways fall short of making the most of our lives.

To be sure, many people are burdened by inappropriate guilt that stems from having unrealistic expectations of themselves or from accepting unrealistic demands from others. When you feel guilty, analyze where those feelings are coming from—have you disappointed yourself in something that is meaningful to you, or are you feeling bad because you are not keeping up with somebody else's expectations? Listen to your guilt—it is cluing you in to act in a manner you know will be more appropriate for you.

BEING INTELLIGENT ABOUT YOUR FEELINGS

You can raise your intelligence by minimizing the influence of disturbing emotions on your thinking and perception. Like any other threat to our security, disturbing emotions can be handled best when we are clear about what we are facing. If you are in a closed room and smell gas, the first thing you do is try to get some ventilation to reduce the toxicity, and then look for the source of the problem so you can eliminate it. Similarly, if disturbing feelings are aroused, first try to reduce their impact by giving yourself a short cooling-off period and then try to determine exactly what it is that is setting off your feelings. Most often you will find that emotions are hard to handle because you are attributing them to the wrong cause. Let's take an example of an emotionally disturbing situation and see how to work with it intelligently.

Suppose you feel very angry when your boss criticizes your work. To react intelligently, you have to get beyond the immediate events that brought the feelings on. Your anger is real, but is it really the boss that is making you angry? At least two possibilities could account for your anger. As you think over the situation it might become clear to you that your work is really quite good and that your boss's criticism is unjustified. You now know that you are angry at the boss for criticizing you unfairly. In this situation the intelligent response is to get back to your boss and review your work together. Suppose, however, that as you go over the situation it becomes clear to you that your work was really quite poor. You are angry at the boss because he aroused your feelings of inadequacy, but you are more angry at yourself for doing a poor job. In this case, the intelligent response is to accept the criticism and use your energy to improve your work.

Let's take another example. Suppose you ask a member of your family to turn down the stereo and that person does so resentfully, making you feel guilty. As you think about the situation, you might come to realize that it was not the stereo that was bothering you but the idea of the listener relaxing while you were busy working. In this case you feel guilty because you were jealous of another person's pleasure. The intelligent response is to provide more enjoyment for yourself. Suppose, however, that as you think about the situation, you realize that the other person always tries to make you feel uncomfortable when you make a request. You feel guilty, all right, but guilty towards yourself that you are not assertive enough in getting what you need. In this case, the intelligent response is to confront the other person about the resentful attitude.

Of course there are many other possible dynamics involved in both of these examples. The point here is primarily to demonstrate an approach for analyzing your feelings in order to respond intelligently.

Exercise _____

Think back to the last emotionally disturbing incident that you were involved in. Now, with paper and pencil, start analyzing it, using the format below.

Situation: Boss criticizes your work.

Emotion Involved	Person Emotion Directed to	Analysis of Situation	Person Really Arousing Emotion	Intelligent Response
Anger	Boss	Work OK, criticism unfair	Boss	Confront boss about work
Anger	Boss	Work poor, boss is right	Self	Improve work performance

Situation: Family member shuts off stereo resentfully.

Emotion Involved	Person Emotion Directed to	Analysis of Situation	Person Really Arousing Emotion	Intelligent Response
Guilt	Family member	Jealous of other's fun	Family member	Enjoy self more
Guilt	Family member	Disturbed at lack of self-assertion	Self	Confront family member

Make a few extra charts for yourself and keep them handy to use when you get upset again. The next time you face an emotionally disturbing situation, get out your chart and analyze the situation. Eventually you will get into the habit of automatically reviewing each emotionally upsetting situation and be able to analyze the causes and respond intelligently.

HIDDEN POWERS OF THE MIND

Our minds function on different levels of consciousness. We are fully aware of some processes, but unaware, or only subliminally aware, of others. Up to now we have talked primarily about increasing intelligence within the framework of our conscious mental functions, but we can also increase intelligence by developing our subconscious mental processes and bringing them into our awareness.

We tend to think of our periods of wakeful consciousness as our highest form of consciousness and the other forms as lower, even labeling them as *sub*conscious or *un*conscious. Actually, it is the other way around. Wakeful consciousness is limited to the information coming to it through the commonly used senses of sight, sound, smell, taste, and touch, and conditioned to process that information through prescribed modes of thought according to culture-bound realities. The subconscious system, which enables us to sense information unavailable through these regular channels and to perceive patterns and meanings not accessible through the constraints of conscious thought, represents a higher form of consciousness and could more appropriately be labeled the *superconscious.*

To bring the neglected aspects of our intelligence into greater play, we have to transcend the conventional perspective of how we function in the world and make ourselves receptive to our subconscious processes.

THE FILTER OF THE MIND

Information about the world comes to us through our sensory systems and we interpret this data to help us make comfortable adaptations to that world. As we saw in the chapter on perception, we manipulate the data to make it more usable: we fill in the blanks and erase or distort the parts that don't seem to make sense. In addition to being unaware of these manipulations, we also tend to be unaware of the full panoply of our sensory systems, acknowledging only the five common ones. The information coming to us from other sensory systems, such as those that monitor our internal states and external energy fields, register only in our subconscious (superconscious) minds. What all this means is that there is a great deal more going on within and without than we are ordinarily conscious of and that for some reason we are programmed to function at a reduced level of awareness. The most plausible theory that has been offered to account for this phenomenon is the filter theory, first proposed by the Nobel laureate Henri Bergson and subsequently accepted by most researchers of the mind. According to this theory, the brain actively screens out stimuli so that the individual is not overwhelmed by sensations. Without a filter, we would be assaulted by more stimulation than we could handle and go on overload. The brain functions as a reducing valve that only allows a small aspect of reality to trickle through to our consciousness, while the remaining aspects stay lodged within our subconscious minds. Turning this around, it also means that we are capable of more heightened perceptions than we ordinarily experience, and that we possess powers of the mind we choose not to use.

Different people have their filters positioned at different points along the sensory continuum. Some are more sensitive to light, some to sound, some to other dimensions. Some open up awareness to new sensory modalities when the old channels are damaged. Blind people, for example, can learn through echolation, a form of sonar, to estimate the size of objects before them and in some way to read color and even large-sized print through a process called derma vision by holding the palms of their hands or their fingertips close to the stimulus. Similarly, different cultures require different sensitivities for optimum adaptation and people in other societies adjust their filters to become more aware of sense modalities we ignore. People in primitive hunting societies are more sensitive to odor than we, and those in primitive agricultural societies are more sensitive to atmospheric stimuli. How we set our filters, and the corresponding view we get of the world, is in good part a matter of value and choice.

In our society, our filters are set to take in information coming from the five common sensory systems, while other sensory input is relegated to the subconscious level. In addition to limiting our awareness to these modalities, we also tend to deny the validity of information processed through other channels. For a long time evidence for the existence of extrasensory perception (ESP) has been denigrated by scientists and the lay public alike because these phenomena flew in the face of what we knew about natural laws. In earlier eras, and in societies with different conceptions about the nature of the world, extrasensory phenomena were accepted as natural manifestations and, accordingly, people relied on these sensory channels for information.

ESP was considered a normal aspect of life until two or three centuries ago. The Greeks regularly consulted with oracles and the Hebrews interpreted dreams to deepen their understanding of the forces operating in the universe. With the Age of Enlightenment and interest in natural science, people became skeptical about ESP experiences, associating them with irrationality and superstition. Studies of primitive societies that escaped enlightenment indicate that many have continued to make extensive use of this source of intelligence. Members of the Senoi tribe in Malaysia, for instance, routinely discuss their dreams each morning to look for guidance in their lives and report to the clan's elders those dreams that have significance for the tribe as a whole. A tribe in New Guinea prepares for visits from distant relatives, which are announced telepathically. Openness to ESP has maintained itself in more highly developed societies too, though among isolated segments of the community, but its occurrence is usually regarded with suspicion, if not derision.

Despite the skepticism towards ESP, the phenomena have refused to go away, and ultimately even the scientists have had to accept the validity of their existence, although unable to account for them. In the late 1800s, the scientific study of psychic phenomena began, under the auspices of the Society for Psychical Research, founded by several leading English scholars. By now so much data has been amassed on the existence of ESP that research emphasis has shifted from merely documenting its appearance to determining how and when it operates.

One of the reasons scientists had difficulty accepting the reality of perceptions that occur outside the realm of ordinary sensory channels was the conceptual barrier created by the theory of behaviorism. B. F. Skinner, the most renowned exponent of this point of view, holds that the mind is a nonexistent entity and that psychic events lack the dimension of physical science.

Interestingly, psychic phenomena have become acceptable to many scientists, not because they have taken on the trappings of physical events, but because physical events have proven to be as amorphous as the psychic ones. New developments in quantum physics have required a reordering of past scientific views about the nature of the physical world and with it the nature of the psychical world. The old laws of space, time, and matter have been replaced by theories about holes in space, time flowing backwards, and negative mass. Within this context, ESP suddenly makes sense and is no stranger than the universe itself. The discovery that matter is at one and the same time both particles and patterns of vibrations makes it perfectly plausible that the physical brain can transmit psychic energy that transcends the bounds of the physical body and can be perceived by outside forces. Because of this coming together of physics and parapsychology, much of the recent work on ESP has been conducted under the auspices of physicists. The theoretical aspects of this work are summarized by Arthur Koestler in his very readable book, *The Roots of Coincidence*, and a review of some of the experimental work on ESP phenomena is provided by the physicist and science writer Charles Panati in *Supersenses*.

With the removal of theoretical barriers to ESP, the major barrier that remains is one of attitude. Many people hesitate to change their focus from the hard data of the physical senses to the finer data of the psychic senses because they fear they may lose their keen analytical abilities. The shift, however, does not require giving up the old way of thinking but adding on a new dimension. Instead of letting so many powers of the mind lie hidden, we can free ourselves to use them when they are appropriate. As we train ourselves to become aware of a broader range of stimuli and information, we still retain the option of when and where we want to apply that skill.

SPLIT CONSCIOUSNESS AND SPLIT BRAIN

Although it is possible to shift our focus of awareness and make the subconscious conscious, we tend to keep these two states of mind segregated from each other. This split, instead of making us clearheaded, actually puts us somewhat at odds with ourselves. When our conscious mind doesn't know what our subconscious is doing, we are just as bemused as when our right hand doesn't know what our left hand is doing. This old saying about the inability to unify the two physical sides of ourselves recognizes a deeper underlying split within our brain. The conscious-subconscious dichotomy, which has also been called a dichotomy between reason and passion, science and art, yang and yin, is reflected in the differences between the left and right hemispheres of the brain.

Your brain is split in two halves—or hemispheres—connected by a thick bundle of nerves called the corpus callosum. It has long been known that each half of the brain controls the opposite half of the body. The left hemisphere controls the right side of the body, and the right hemisphere controls the left side of the body. Differences between the two hemispheres were first noted over a hundred years ago by Paul Broca. In postmortem dissections of the brains of patients who had been unable to speak, he found severe damage in what is now called Broca's area, a small area on the left frontal lobe. Another surgeon, Karl Wernicke, found another language center in the left hemisphere that controlled the ability to understand language, either spoken or written. Subsequent research on patients with damage to the right side of the brain found that they were unable to recognize people and things, sometimes even their own face in the mirror.

In the 1950s, further discoveries on the nature of the differences between the right and left hemispheres were made after the introduction of split-brain surgery, which involves severing the corpus callosum. This surgery was done on epileptic patients in order to control the spread of seizures from one side of the brain to the other. The operation results in the inability of the right and left hemispheres to communicate with each other; information reaching one side of the brain cannot then transfer to the other. From studies on patients with split-brain surgery, it was possible to determine more clearly the functions of each half of the brain. Dr. Roger Sperry, a brain scientist who spearheaded research in this area and was recently awarded a Nobel prize for his work on hemisphere functions, found that the left hemisphere, in addition to being the verbal hemisphere, operates in a logical, analytical, computerlike fashion. It processes information serially, or one piece after the other. In contrast, the right hemisphere is specialized for visual and spatial thinking, dealing with complex patterns. Instead of dealing sequentially with information bit by bit, it processes stimuli simultaneously, at any given moment organizing information into one unified whole. In more specific terms, the left side of the brain does our reading, writing, and arithmetic, but the right side does our singing, fantasizing, and dreaming. Dr. Robert Ornstein, a neuropsychologist, describes the right hemisphere as the silent side and mode of the night. According to Ornstein, it is the right side that enables us to be open to extrasensory communication.

In our culture, left-brain functions are valued over right-brain functions and given disproportionate attention in the educational system. Children are taught the three Rs and how to think logically, but are discouraged from engaging in fantasy. Music, art, dance, and other imaginative activities are relegated to extracurricular status. This results in a widespread tendency for left-brain dominance, which is manifested by the many right-handed people you see. Although our left-brain functions are clearly necessary, so are our right-brain functions. When we rely on the left hemisphere to the exclusion of the right, we are really acting like half-wits, letting important faculties of the mind go to waste. Truly intelligent behavior requires a harmonious balance of the two mentations.

OPENING THE DOORS
TO YOUR SUPERCONSCIOUS

Several factors play a role in developing your receptivity to a wider range of sensory information and your ability to bring more of it to your awareness. A very basic factor is your belief in the possibility of doing so, since our beliefs determine our experience and become self-fulfilling prophecies. The brief review of the origin and nature of your hidden mental powers we have presented was intended, in part, to help you see what is available to you. Try not to reject the possibilities of your mind just because they might seem strange and incomprehensible right now.

In cultures where there is no philosophic barrier to accepting the validity of expanded awareness and ESP phenomena, such awareness does occur. Similarly, people who believe in the possibility of making contact with the psychic energy field are, in fact, the ones who become psychic. A person's attitude to his or her own abilities in this regard is a crucial determinant of how successful one can be. Experiments have shown that most people respond telepathically to transmitted information above what could be expected by mere chance. Professor Gertrude Schmeidler, a psychologist and psychic researcher, also found that persons who strongly disbelieve in the possibility of ESP perform significantly below chance expectation in telepathy experiments—they succeed at failing. Schmeidler concluded that their excessive failures seemed like "an unconscious avoidance of the correct response—which of course implies some unconscious information about it." In a subsequent experiment, Schmeidler found that the difference between the above-chance scores of those who accepted the possibility of their success at ESP and the below-chance scores of those who rejected this possibility was significant at odds of less than a million to one.

A second factor influencing receptivity is intention. If you want to develop your hidden mental powers and extrasensory perceptions, you must also develop the intention to do so. To help you in exerting your will, make clear to yourself what your reasons are for wanting to cultivate your extrasensory capacities. Intention, however, is not enough; a lot of effort and practice will also be required; but they, too, are fueled by intention.

Another important factor in bringing more sensory information into your awareness is your ability to shift your focus of attention from the usual sensory channels. When we are in a wake state, we usually give our full attention to information coming to us through the five common sensory systems. We all experience what happens when attention is withdrawn from those systems, which happens every time we fall asleep. At those times, our mental processes, instead of being directed outward and in their usual state of vigilance, are directed inward and are more relaxed. Accompanying this change in direction goes a corresponding change in the nature of our experience. Although our bodies are asleep, our minds are not asleep, but actively engaged in a different sort of consciousness known as dreaming. In contrast to the logical thought characteristic of waking consciousness, dreams are characterized by vivid sensory images, in which events flow in nonrational and nonlinear fashion.

The same alteration of consciousness that we experience during sleep also occurs in other states in which attention is withdrawn from the usual sensory channels. In the drowsy period just before sleep, as we start to turn off outside stimuli, we experience hypnagogic images—those rich visual images that succeed each other in disconnected fashion. During intense religious, aesthetic, and intellectual experiences our mind is so engrossed that we dissociate from ordinary sensations and thereby enter a state of expanded consciousness.

In addition to these spontaneous shifts of attention from the usual sensory channels, we can try to shift attention deliberately to attain an altered state of consciousness. A common way is through rhythmic stimulation. Music helps to shut out other stimuli and to redirect attention to its harmonies and rhythms, allowing alterations in consciousness to occur, which is why it is so widely used in religious rituals, tribal rites, and discotheques. A shift in sensory focus has also been sought through use of mushrooms, peyote, mescaline, marijuana, and LSD. While such substances do succeed in helping us to remove our mental filters and to achieve expanded awareness, they can also have dangerous immediate and long-range consequences and, in fact, have given altered states of consciousness a bad reputation.

Of all the deliberate routes for shifting our focus and achieving higher levels of consciousness, relaxation exercises and meditation are the most practical, safest, and potentially most beneficial methods. We have already described relaxation techniques in the chapter on emotions. In the next section we will discuss meditation.

Before moving on, we want to emphasize that altered states of consciousness are a natural manifestation and an important avenue to realizing our full potential. If you want to obtain a broader understanding of the role that altered states can play in our lives, read Lawrence LeShan's book, *Alternate Realities*.

HOW TO MEDITATE

Meditation, while relatively new in the West, has a centuries-old tradition in the East existing in somewhat different forms among the Yogis of India, the Buddhists of China, the Zen Buddhists of Japan, and the Sufis of the Middle East. The meditator tries to discipline the mind in order to achieve release from the constraints of conscious awareness, thereby achieving oneness with the universe. According to these systems, the mind under ordinary circumstances is constantly assaulted by stimuli; the essential power that resides inside the individual cannot surface in this chaos. When one can free oneself from these bombardments both physically and psychologically, one can then enter into direct communication with nature, of which one is a part. The meditator's consciousness is thus not closed off, but expanded.

The meditator seeks to quiet the body and reduce the impact of stimuli through mental concentration. Experimental studies on persons during meditation indicate that this shifting away from ordinary sensory experience alters not only the meditator's subjective experience, but the whole metabolic system as well. During meditation, oxygen consumption is sharply curtailed; carbon dioxide elimination falls off; blood pressure, heart rate, and lactate level in the blood (which is associated with anxiety) decrease; and skin resistance to electrical current increases, as do the slow alpha rhythms of the brain. These signs together indicate a person who is at a high level of relaxation and calm. The machinery of the body is, as it were, allowed to rest, enabling the mind to move its attention inward.

Meditation is taught at many yoga institutes and at the popular Transcendental Meditation society. You can also learn to meditate on your own. The technique is simple, but it requires patience and persistence, and the most important determinant of your success will be your determination to make it work.

In order to meditate, you need a quiet environment, an object to dwell on, and about thirty minutes of undisturbed time. Choose a room that you find congenial, with a flow of fresh air, and make sure that once you start there will be no interferences until you have finished the session. Wear comfortable, loose clothing.

To start your session, seat yourself in a comfortable position. Some people prefer a straight chair with feet flat on the floor and hands in the lap. Some prefer to sit on the floor with legs crossed in what is called the *lotus position*. If you are not accustomed to this position, stick with the chair, so you remain comfortable throughout your session. Do not lie down, because you might fall asleep.

Meditation consists of concentration. An easy way to begin is by concentrating on an object, or a sound. If you choose an object, anything will do, provided it is pleasant and has neutral connotations for you. Some people use a flower, some a picture, some a candle flame. Place the object so that you can gaze at it steadily without strain or discomfort. Look at it with your full attention, but do not stare. Try to be totally involved in seeing the object. If your mind should start to wander, fix your attention back on the object. Give yourself over totally to looking.

If you choose to meditate on a sound, or mantra, choose a word or phrase that you find compatible. Some people prefer a meaningless phrase, like *Da-dum*, some prefer an ancient chant like *Om* and some prefer a simple word like *Peace*. One of the rationales for using a mantra is that mouthing the chant sets up vibrations in the body that help you achieve a higher state of consciousness. The purpose of having a guru choose your mantra is, supposedly, that the chosen mantra will resonate in tune with your personal rhythms, but you can experiment by yourself to determine which sound feels good to you. Once you have selected your sound, start chanting it aloud, at a slow but steady pace. Just keep chanting, involving yourself more and more. As with meditation on an object, the purpose of meditation on a sound is to keep you concentrating on just that one activity. Chant, and be aware only of your chanting.

That, simply, is the meditation process. As you focus on your object or your sound, fill yourself with this and nothing else. Empty your mind of all thoughts, emotions and physical sensations. Do not strain and do not be concerned about how well you are doing. When your mind wanders—and it will do a lot of that at first—do not get upset with yourself, but redirect your attention back to your object or sound. Take your time and don't be self-critical. The important thing is not how well you do, but that you persist in doing it.

Once you start meditating, it is important that you have a session at least once every day, and twice a day is better. The best times are early in the morning or late afternoon or evening. One should not meditate for two hours after a meal, since the digestive process seems to interfere. The length of time is not as important as the regularity; for most people twenty to thirty minutes is enough.

USING YOUR DREAMS

Dreams are one form of extrasensory perception that is available to us nightly, but only few of us make significant use of what we see. In the dream state, as in states induced by meditation, the body is at rest, the metabolic system is slowed down, and the sense organs are relaxed, allowing the mind to move out and beyond the self. Although we have become used to thinking about dream material in Freudian terms as an expression of our unconscious, there is just as much if not more reason to view dreams as an expression of our superconscious reaching out far beyond the self, rather than merely further back into the self.

We are all familiar with the precognitive dreams reported in the Bible, whether of Pharoah and the seven fat and lean cows, of Joseph and the sheaves of wheat, or of Pontius Pilate's wife. Similarly, many of us have either had our own precognitive dreams or heard about those of others, either our acquaintances or people of renown. There are also telepathic dreams, which inform us of current happenings and are just as frequent, if not as dramatic. Telepathic dreams have also been produced under controlled experimental conditions. In the famous dream laboratory at the Maimonides Medical Center, Dr. Montague Ullman and Dr. Stanley Krippner had people check in at their usual bedtime and go to sleep in the dream chamber, wired to delicate machinery to monitor their brain waves and rapid eye movements (REMs). In a separate room, another person, the sender, sat alone with a collection of sealed envelopes, each containing a reproduction of a well-known painting. As the experiment began, the sender opened the envelopes randomly during the course of the night and looked at them one at a time, concentrating on sending each picture to the dreamer. The dreamer was awakened by the experimenters each time there was a lot of dream activity, as indicated by the REMs, and asked to report on what he or she was dreaming. In the morning, tapes of the dream reports and the pictures were given to a panel of judges, who had to determine the degree of correspondence between them. Data from these studies, amassed over a period of many years and with many subjects, indicate that telepathic dreams are a reality.

Our dreams inform us in yet another way. They sometimes enable us to reach understandings about problems that elude us during our wake state. We have already discussed the intuitive dream of Kekule, who was able to solve a difficult chemistry problem in his dream. Others, as well, find that dreams provide insights and solutions they cannot attain in normal consciousness, when their thinking is confined to stricter verbal, logical modes. The widespread use of dreams in psychotherapy attests to the help that dreams can provide in offering us solutions to emotional problems. Dreams are also a source of artistic inspiration. The story of "Dr. Jekyll and Mr. Hyde" came to Robert Louis Stevenson in one of his dreams and Bram Stoker conceived of Dracula through a nightmare.

The first step in using the information supplied by your dreams is to become more aware of the dreams that you have. Although many people maintain they hardly ever dream, research in the dream laboratories has clearly established that everyone dreams every night and, moreover, has several dream periods within one night. The best way to remember your dreams is to develop the conscious intent that you will do so. When you go to bed at night, tell yourself that you are going to remember your dreams, and when you wake up, whether in the middle of the night or in the morning, be sure that you immediately record your dreams. You can either jot them down (keep a pad and pencil handy for that purpose) or keep a tape recorder at your bedside. After a while, remembering your dreams will become habitual.

Once you have your dreams recorded, the next step is interpreting them. Since dreams are the product of an altered state of consciousness, they speak in the language of that state. This is not the logical, verbal language of our wake state, but a vivid and image-rich language that does not follow sequential rules. Again, our Freudian heritage does us a disservice in suggesting that the strange and sometimes illogical images are intended to conceal the truth from us when, instead, they are trying to reveal the truth to us. According to Carl Jung, the Swiss psychoanalyst, our dreams also put us in touch with the collective unconscious, the pooled knowledge of the species, which speaks to us in universally shared symbols.

Dream images can best be regarded as poetic metaphors that are trying to clarify aspects of life that go beyond the capacity of mere language to express. Do not be concerned that all your images are expressing repressed fantasies of your unconscious mind. Remember, instead, that they are expressing more universal truths of your superconscious mind. Many dream books offer guides to dream interpretation, supplying you with meanings that various dream objects are supposed to connote. Do not get stuck on rigid interpretations and stay close to what you know about the images you dreamed of. Some books suggest, for instance, that all elongated objects you dream about, such as a snake, skyscraper, or rifle, signify a penis. Even though a snake, skyscraper, and rifle all are long objects, they also represent important differences: one is a living creature, one a lifeless edifice, and one an instrument of destruction. Kekule's snake, as we saw before, was not a sex organ but a metaphor for organic structure. If you let your dream images speak for themselves, their meaning will become apparent.

TRAINING YOUR ESP FACULTIES

In the following pages we will be discussing how to develop extrasensory capacities. We have included those psychic powers that expand your awareness of the environment—telepathy, psychometry, clairvoyance, and auric reading—but not those that are more oriented towards affecting the environment, such as psychokinesis and healing.

Developing your psychic powers requires confidence in the possibility that you can make this happen. If you do not already have that confidence, we suggest you first read more about ESP to become familiar with the research evidence and to learn about other people's experiences and the types of phenomena they have encountered. Many books are available on this subject and some are included in the suggested reading list. In addition to confidence, your training will require a lot of time and patience. You will be calling forth aspects of the brain that have been dormant for most of your life, and they will take a while to awaken and stabilize. Even when aroused relatively quickly, your ESP faculties need training to become reliable and capable of producing meaningful results.

When you start your training, it will be facilitated by setting up suitable conditions beforehand to help put you in a receptive frame of mind. Follow the steps outlined each time you have a training session.

Preparing the Environment

Set aside a block of time in which you will not be disturbed. Use a room that is warm but not stuffy, dimly lit, and insulated from noise and outside interferences.

Have a tape recorder or assistant available so you can keep a complete record of your sessions. Try to get into the habit of verbalizing your impressions out loud so that you will have a verbatim transcript. Many of your impressions will be fleeting ones and apt to get lost if not recorded. It is difficult to appreciate the significance of your impressions while they are coming in and some seemingly minor ones may, in retrospect, be more important than you immediately realized. If you feel awkward about recording yourself, practice free-associating out loud to the tape recorder before you begin your ESP training. After a while this will seem perfectly natural to you and you will be able to record your ESP session without feeling as if there is an intrusive presence that might block your impressions.

Before the session, make notes regarding all outside influences, such as weather, atmospheric conditions, phases of the moon, and so on. Certain conditions are more conducive to ESP than others, and you may find different rates of success depending on these external factors. Variations in your mood also have an effect and should be noted.

Preparing Yourself

Practice only when you feel emotionally calm and not beset by problems. People occasionally have spontaneous ESP experiences when they are under stress, but it is best to avoid practicing at such times. If you are emotionally upset, there is a possibility that some of your ESP impressions can disturb you further and, should that happen, you might find it difficult to shut off the influx of impressions when you want to.

Seat yourself comfortably and loosen up any restrictive clothing you might be wearing.

Always start your sessions with a serious commitment to work and the intention to receive psychic information (or send it). Begin your sessions with a relaxation exercise.

HOW TO PRACTICE TELEPATHY

Telepathy is the direct communication of impressions from one mind to another, independent of the recognized sensory channels. Of all psychic phenomena, telepathy is the easiest for people to accept because it is a natural extension of our usual modes of communication. In addition to listening to people when they speak, we have learned how to read their moods and thoughts through their body language and, with those to whom we are close, we can pick up subtle nuances of feeling even without this visible information. It has long been part of the folklore that a mother can sense when her infant is in distress, even though at the other end of the house, and this has been documented in Soviet studies of mother-infant telepathy. Mothers at an obstetrics clinic were kept in one wing of a building and their babies in another yet, when blood samples were taken from the babies, the mothers showed measurable signs of anxiety. Twins have also been known to have strong telepathic bonds. One of the most dramatic instances on record involved Betty Jo Eller and Bobbie Jean Eller, identical twins from North Carolina. Throughout childhood they were inseparable, always mirroring each other, even to the extent of becoming sick together. In adulthood, when one became schizophrenic the other did too, but when hospitalized they were separated and placed in different wings of the building. On the night Bobbie Jean had a catatonic seizure and died, the staff checked the ward where Betty Jo was kept and found her dead, lying in exactly the same position as her twin sister.

In the ordinary course of a day, we probably receive many telepathic communications, but because of their unsensational nature are not aware that they are telepathic. We tend to take notice only of those communications associated with strong emotional messages, such as are involved in traumatic incidents. E. Douglas Dean, an engineer and psychical researcher, has experimentally demonstrated that people receive telepathic messages of which they are not consciously aware. He had the people who were sending the messages (*senders*) and those receiving (*receivers*) seated in different rooms. The senders were given a stack of cards, each bearing the name of a person; some names were drawn at random from the phone book and some belonged to people emotionally close to the receiver. The sender concentrated on transmitting one name at a time to the receiver. When the sender was concentrating on the name of a person emotionally close to the receiver, the latter, though not consciously aware of receiving a telepathic communication, showed significant changes in finger blood volume, a characteristic of emotional reactions. This and other experiments suggest that a lot of the changes in our mood during the day that we cannot account for reflect the unconscious reception of such telepathic messages.

To practice telepathy, you will need a partner to take turns acting as receiver and sender with you. It is important to work with someone with whom you are emotionally compatible, as that will affect your ability to transmit well to each other. You will need two additional persons to act as assistants. Basically, your practice sessions will consist of the sender's trying to transmit a picture to the receiver. Use pictures that are interesting and vivid, capable of arousing emotions as well as sensations of taste, touch, and so on. Try sessions of up to ten transmissions at a time and don't compare notes to evaluate hits or misses until your session is over. Be prepared, initially, for a rate of failure that is much greater than the rate of success.

Have the sender seated comfortably at a table on which is placed the picture or object to be transmitted. The sender should be able to look at the picture without any strain. The assistant's role is to present pictures (or objects) to the sender, and to keep careful notes of the time each picture is presented, as well as of any other relevant data (light flashing through window, etc.) The sender should start by asserting to him- or herself the intention to transmit the picture. The sender has to form a clear visual image of the picture to be sent. Concentration on the picture without visualization does not work, since it is the visualization that is transmitted. The sender has to create as complete an image as possible, including the emotions, scent and textures involved, while maintaining a relaxed, nonstraining attitude, and imagining the receiver to be very close by. Transmit for twenty to thirty seconds at most.

It is important that the receiver spends the first five seconds deliberately reaching out to the sender with the intention of receiving the transmission. After that, the receiver should sit back comfortably and wait for impressions. During practice, any impressions received, whether major or minor, whether tactile, auditory, olfactory, or visual, should be described by the receiver and recorded and timed by the assistant. Although the sender will be transmitting for only about thirty seconds, up to fifteen minutes must be allowed for the receiver to record impressions, as they usually take time to seep through to consciousness. In between transmissions, it is a good idea for the receiver to get up and walk around a bit.

As mentioned, it is unlikely that you will have much success on your first tries, but that does not mean that you cannot develop your telepathic powers. It takes time and effort to develop this capacity, just as it does any other skill. There are also many outside factors that can influence your success. Some people work better together than others, and you may want to experiment with different partners. In addition to the messages that you are intentionally trying to receive, keep in mind that you may be the recipient of other messages that you are not soliciting. Even your assistants may be unknowingly transmitting to you during the time of your session. So don't be too quick to dismiss the results you obtain.

HOW TO PRACTICE PSYCHOMETRY

Psychometry is the ability to acquire information through the mind about an object held in one's hand. The desire for psychometric ability is commonly expressed, although unwittingly, when people hold a valued object in their hands and say, "Oh, if only this could talk." Actually, objects do talk to people, even though the impressions received may be dismissed. Not infrequently, for example, people receive dim emotional impressions or visions when touching antiques or heirlooms. Although it may seem far out to you to think that you can receive impressions just through touch, remember that touch is the most basic of your senses, from which the others evolved. In addition to the common but unacknowledged experiences of psychometry are well-documented experiences of psychics who work with various police units throughout the country to find missing persons. These psychics locate people by "reading" objects belonging to the lost party.

Despite the fact that we know it occurs, psychometry appears to us to be a strange phenomenon that is hard to accept. The best theory to date to account for its occurrence is that the basic substance underlying matter contains the memory of everything it has come in contact with and that this, in turn, is available to the psychometrist. In the East, this concept is known and accepted as the *Akashic Record*, or *Cosmic Memory*.

Two preparatory steps are necessary for psychometry. One is the sharpening of your observational faculties and the other is the development of your descriptive faculties. The reason you want to develop these faculties is that impressions can come flooding in en masse and if you have not honed your observational abilities, you may miss out both on detail and order of sequence, which could lead to distorted impressions. Similarly, if you are not adept at describing your impressions, the record you make will also appear distorted. The exercises outlined in the chapter on perception for utilizing your olfactory, tactile, auditory, and gustatory senses are all good practice for increasing your observational powers. You can also use your time sitting on the bus or waiting in line at the supermarket to create visual images of your best friend's face, with attention given to the hairline, hair texture, shape of brow, furrows on the brow, eyebrows, eyelids, shape of eyes, and so on. In this same fashion, you can practice visualizing any other person or object you know. Picture an orange in your mind, notice its overall shape, look at the indentations in the skin, observe the top where the stem attaches, scratch the peel with your fingernail and see yourself bringing the orange to your nose, then smell the aroma of the orange oils. When you describe your impressions, similarly, try to recreate their richness by going over them methodically and in full detail.

Another important preparatory step in psychometry is to prepare yourself to listen attentively to your impressions, but to stay emotionally disengaged. It is possible for some objects, because of their histories, to arouse negative feelings on your part. If you cannot stay detached, you might find yourself swamped with your feelings and losing contact with the psychic impressions.

In choosing an object for psychometry practice, you will need someone who knows it well to prepare a full history of it. Each object has both a personal history and a gathered history, the former being impressions that belong to it inherently and the other being the sum of impressions of the people who have been involved with it. For training purposes, it is best if you can use objects owned only by one person, so that your impressions are easier to organize. Keys, for instance, are poor objects for beginners, since they usually pass through many hands, whereas jewelry often has had only one owner and is usually easier to work with. Letters are also good objects for beginning psychometry, as are ribbons, ties, and other personal objects.

To start your practice session, take the object in your hand or, if you prefer, hold it lightly to your forehead. Close your eyes and assume a receptive mental state, waiting calmly for impressions. If you feel a physical reaction, or if you have negative feelings about the object, put it down and try again with another object. When you practice you might be more successful if, after a time, you ask for information rather than just wait for it to come. Formulate questions to the object that can be answered in simple pictorial terms.

At first, your ratio of hits to misses will be quite low but, again, do not let this discourage you. Even if only one of your impressions is valid, that is a good start. By going over your records, you will be able to track the conditions under which you seem to do better; you can try to adjust your practice sessions accordingly.

DEVELOPING AURIC SIGHT

All living things have an aura or halo around them. Although not ordinarily visible to the eye, the aura can be photographed by a process developed in the Soviet Union, known as Kirlian photography, after its inventors Semyon and Valentina Kirlian. Just what the aura consists of is still not entirely clear, but there is general agreement that it is a field of force emanating from living matter that exists in direct proportion to the life processes occurring within. The idea of a basic life force is not new and has existed in many cultures under many names: *prana, ka, mana, ch'i,* and, more recently, *bioplasma.* When living things die and the life force dissipates, their auras fade and finally disappear; when they are alive, the peaks and color reflect the health and energy level of the person, animal, or plant. The halos of mythical and biblical figures suggest, in light of current understanding, that people who reportedly had auras were possessed of an exceptionally powerful life force and/or that in other eras people were more attuned to perceiving the auras that we now know surround all living things.

The aura forms an oval shape around the body and looks as if it is made of fine hairs. It consists of a dark area, of up to ¼-inch thickness, which exactly follows the outline of the body, an inner aura that follows the general shape of the body and is about four inches from its surface, and an outer aura that extends to about twelve inches from the body. Under some circumstances, still another finer aura can be seen, which extends out indefinitely.

When a person is in good health, the surface of the aura is unbroken. People who are not well appear to have tears in the aura where, supposedly, vital energy can leak out. These tears are located at the point of injury or disease. It has been demonstrated, through the Kirlian process, that psychic healing involves an interchange of energy from healer to patient such that the patient's aura registers an increase in width and repair at the tears, while the healer's aura shows a corresponding decrease in size after treatment.

There are two ways to develop your auric sight—by touch and by vision. You will need some volunteers to make their bodies available to you for auric reading. Also have available outline drawings of the body from front and side views on which you can record your impressions. When taking your reading your subject can either sit up or lie down.

To read by touch, pass your hands slowly downwards over the body, keeping your hands two to three inches from the body and never touching. Focus your attention on your fingertips and on the different sensations you feel as you move your hands further away from the body and closer in. Do not be discouraged if you feel nothing at first. It may take you a long time before you can attune yourself to the fine emanations of the aura. When you do experience them, they will have a vibrant feel that may be either cold or warm. When this experience occurs, move your hands out and try to feel how far the aura extends as well as any variations in its contour. Sketch the aura to help in your perception of it. When you have been able to trace the inner aura with your hands, you can then move on to the outer aura, holding your hands at a distance of about a foot.

To read the aura visually, have your subject wear a leotard or tight-fitting clothes and stand against a dark wall. Do not stare at the person but, rather, try to put your eyes slightly out of focus by focusing on a point roughly six inches beyond. Do not strain, but look at your subject in a relaxed manner. When you see the aura, it will look like a luminous haze around the body. Once you are able to perceive this, try to view the whole aura and note any deviations in its shape. Have your subject change positions so you can try to see the aura from different perspectives.

As with the practice of the other extrasensory modes, be patient and do not expect quick results. This is a new way of perceiving for you, which will take time and persistence to develop.

When you become more adept at reading the aura, you will be able to notice variations in the color. Since the color of a person's aura can vary depending on his or her health and emotional state, interpretations based on color should not be made on the basis of only one reading. The color of the aura is a guide to the character and temperament of the person. Although standard interpretations of the various colors have been made, it is better that you work with aura colors as with dream images—making interpretations that seem most meaningful to you. The whole purpose of reading an aura is to develop your own intuitive and extrasensory faculties and your interpretations are just a part of that process.

DEVELOPING CLAIRVOYANT SKILLS

Clairvoyance is the ability to perceive events hidden from ordinary senses; it includes precognition, or the perception of events yet to occur. Although it is easier for most of us to conceptualize the possibility of making contact with events of the past, anecdotal reports of precognitive experiences are much more frequent. The new discoveries in physics, however, have made the phenomenon of precognition more understandable, since the progression of time now appears to be merely a subjective experience that has no objective significance. As Einstein wrote, the separation of past, present, and future is "mere illusion."

History abounds with stories of precognition, including those of the Greek oracles and of Joseph in Egypt. We have all heard of people having precognitive visions, usually of some catastrophic event, and such experiences have been recorded by researchers in the tens of thousands. Dreams are a particularly good medium for precognition. Probably America's most famous precognitive dreamer was Abraham Lincoln. Being a very skeptical man, he was unsettled by the power of his dreams' messages, but he took them seriously nevertheless. Lincoln's dreams foretold of his rise to power and sudden death at the height of his career. A week before his assassination, he had a prophetic dream of his funeral, which he witnessed in detail, including the corpse in the East Room.

The experiments in the laboratory are much less interesting but, nonetheless, demonstrate clearly the existence of precognitive abilities, even among animals. Mice and hamsters, for example, have been placed in a two-compartment cage with an electrified wire floor, which emitted mild charges to one or the other compartment at random. The animals were free to move from compartment to compartment to avoid being shocked, if they could intuit which compartment would be charged. Both hamsters and mice have demonstrated high rates of precognition, being able to avoid the compartments about to be charged. Similar experiments have been tried with humans, although without the shock, and they have performed as well, being able to predict, above chance, the occurrence of random events. Dr. Helmut Schmidt, a physicist interested in psychic research, designed an experiment in which subjects had to predict which one of four colored lights would go on. The lights were activated by the decay of radioactive material, a totally random occurrence. Although no one, including the experimenter, had any way of predicting which atoms would decay and thereby, which light would be activated, the average results with sensitive subjects ran from odds against chance success of two billion to one to over ten billion to one.

Clairvoyant practice does not require any assistants and you can do it by yourself. Make sure you eat only a light meal before a session, however, or you might fall asleep. In training your clairvoyant powers, you will be projecting outwardly whatever visual impressions you receive. To do this, you need some surface on which to project. This is where the idea of crystal balls developed. If you have a crystal ball, by all means use it. Place it on a black cloth and be careful to not let light shine on it. If you do not have one, you can just as easily use a bowl filled with black ink or cut yourself out a five-inch circle of black matte paper and mount it on a white cardboard. Sit comfortably at a table so that you can rest your eyes easily on whatever projecting surface you are using.

To begin your session, look at the surface in a relaxed way. You will probably find that it shifts in and out of focus and that you develop an itch at the tip of your nose or between your eyes. Try to disregard these sensations and keep looking, being careful not to strain. For your first few sessions you may not experience anything more than the itch and shift of focus. At your following sessions, if you maintain a relaxed state, you will start to see a mist with occasional sparks of light. You may also see fleeting images that last for a second or two. These are not clairvoyant images but similar to the hypnagogic images you see in the drowsy period just before the onset of sleep. These images indicate that you are in a receptive state. Stay prepared yet calm, because excitement will drive further images away.

As you continue to look at the projecting surface you will see other images, which linger. These will be a combination of ordinary everyday things as well as things that appear in unfamiliar and symbolic form. These latter images will have to be interpreted, as in dreams, and may be accompanied by strong emotional feelings, which will help you in understanding them better. Usually the images that come to you with a clear sense of their meaning are providing you with correct information. The more uncertain you are, the further away your interpretation is from the real meaning that is trying to communicate itself.

When you are finished with your session, make sure you announce this to yourself in order to shut off the flow of images. It is important that you maintain control over your clairvoyant visions, only working with them at times you intentionally designate. If you become adept at clairvoyance and do not take this precaution, you could find yourself involuntarily swamped by your psychic impressions.

THE CARE AND FEEDING OF YOUR BRAIN

Your brain is the most important organ in your body. It not only is the control center that keeps the rest of you functioning but it also makes you distinctively *you*. Although you could probably imagine what your life would be like after a heart transplant, chances are you can't begin to imagine what it would be like to have a brain transplant. Despite its central importance, people pay little attention to their brains. They worry about their hearts and cholesterol intake or their lungs and cigarette smoking, but who cares about his or her brain? The major reason for this blasé attitude is that people do not realize that the health of their brain can vary according to the treatment it receives. Knowing what to eat, what not to eat, and how to exercise your brain can keep it in top-notch physical condition and working at its optimum. This chapter offers you a summary of the information currently available on maintaining the health of your brain. But first, let's take a closer look at how your brain works.

SOME SHOCKING FACTS ABOUT YOUR BRAIN

Like other organs in your body, your brain is composed of cells. Unlike the cells of other organs, however, brain cells, called neurons, will not regenerate if damaged. If a portion of your liver is removed, new liver tissue will grow to replace it, with the cells of the remaining tissue dividing until the original size of the liver is restored. If a neuron dies, that's it. It is not replaced by another, and no cell division takes place. Fortunately, we come equipped with an impressive number of neurons, conservatively estimated at 15 billion (roughly the same number as there are stars in the Milky Way). But it is also estimated that between 1,000 to 100,000 of these neurons die every day, depending on your age. Some brain researchers take comfort in the fact that given so many brain cells to start with, this loss represents only a small percent of the total. Looked at from a slightly different point of view, you can unnecessarily lose between one to two billion brain cells in a lifetime—vital brain power gone to waste. This loss occurs not through accident or trauma, but simply through lack of proper care.

The intelligence at your disposal is related to the number of brain cells you have. Human intelligence has evolved far beyond that of other animals primarily because of the growth in brain size and the accompanying increase in brain cells, particularly in the cortex. Humans have larger brains in relation to body size than most other animals, and they have a higher number of cortical neurons in relation to body weight. But the number of neurons is only half the story. Intelligence also depends on the interconnections these neurons make with one another. It is the circuits established among brain cells that make for usable intelligence. These connections, called synapses, allow signals to pass from cell to cell, making it possible for the brain to code, classify, and operate on information coming in from diverse sources.

While the number of neurons is set at birth, the number of connections among brain cells keeps on growing. Most researchers conservatively estimate the number of possible brain cell connections at 10,000 per neuron, although brain cells with connections to 20,000 other brain cells have been discovered. Even at the lower figure, this means each person is capable of forming a minimum of 10 trillion connections among brain cells, or 30,000 times more connections than the number of people in the world. Yet, despite the vast possibilities our brains have to offer, very little use is made of them. Of the 10,000 connections possible for each neuron, most people establish only about 100! This paltry development of brain potential results primarily from lack of stimulation. Even those connections that have been formed will maintain their efficiency only through continued use and proper care.

THE KEY TO
HEALTHY CELLS AND CIRCUITS

How do you establish the cell connections that are the basis of intelligence, and how do you keep your brain cells from dying?

Ideally, care of your brain should start before you are born. The brain is in the process of formation and growth in the embryonic and fetal stages, and any nutritional deficiency at these times, or the presence of toxic substances, can hamper the development of a healthy brain. At birth, as already mentioned, the brain has all its cells, and is closer to its adult development than any other organ, taking up 10 percent of body weight. This is why babies have such big heads in relation to body size. The rest of the body still has to grow, but the brain is basically all there. Most of the brain development after birth involves glial cells, which take care of food and waste transport and provide insulation.

A sound nutritional and toxin-free environment is as vital to the brain after birth as before, but stimulation is just as important. Food keeps the brain cells healthy and external stimulation goads them into making contact. Children who are deprived of essential nutrition can suffer irreversible brain damage and the accompanying retardation. Approximately 300 million children are so affected. Even proper feeding, though, is not sufficient to keep children's intellectual functioning up to par. Children who are brought up in institutions where they are given adequate diets but inadequate stimulation and handling by adults are slow to develop and remain apathetic. Not only is cultural deprivation known to lower one's intellectual functioning level, but the obverse has also been demonstrated. As we described in the first chapter, children reared in homes where there is a lot of stimulation and challenge develop into brighter and seemingly more intelligent people. Thus first-born children, who receive more parental attention than their siblings, tend to be the higher achievers.

It is, of course, difficult to demonstrate how nutrition and stimulation actually alter the health and complexity of the brain, since that organ is not ordinarily available for inspection. Most studies infer brain condition from behavior, but some data is available through brain autopsies on children who have died in infancy. Such studies reveal that with undernourishment, the brain is smaller than normal and there are fewer glial cells. Studies on animals also demonstrate the lack of brain development that results from insufficient nourishment and stimulation. A study on rats showed that enriching their environment (from being reared in solitary confinement compared to being reared with other rats in a cage with stimulating toys) led to an increase in the number of brain cells, the number of connecting fibers, and cortical weight.

To understand why nutrition is so important, let's take a look at what actually goes on in your head. Brain cells connect with each other by means of shoots known as axons and dendrites. The axons, long fibers extending from the cell body, transmit signals to other neurons. The dendrites, short fibers that branch out from the cell, pick up impulses being transmitted by neighboring cells. Axons and dendrites do not actually touch each other, and the nerve impulse must jump across the gap (synapse) between them. Nerve impulses travel through the neuron electrically, but they are transmitted over the synapse biochemically by substances known as neurotransmitters. As the electrical signal strikes the terminal buttons of the axon, tiny sacs burst open, spilling out neurotransmitters that flow across the synaptic gap, touching the dendrites of the adjacent cell, and sparking an electric current. The ability to make neuronal connections and, therefore, the intelligence at your disposal, depends on the biochemical balance of your body.

Brain cells need a constant supply of nourishment and oxygen to keep healthy and do their work. The neurons require energy and nutrients both to synthesize the proteins needed for impulse transmission, and to transport this material. Each neuron transports roughly three times its own volume daily. Although only 2 percent to 3 percent of total body weight, the brain consumes 25 percent of the body's oxygen intake. The brain is protected against shortages of essential nutrients by a process called brain sparing, which ensures that the brain gets its supplies before the other organs. But, if continued undernourishment occurs, the brain is also shortchanged. Roughly 1½ pints of blood flow through the brain every minute, carrying oxygen and food. Just a five-second interruption in this blood flow can render a person unconscious, and if the interruption lasts just a few minutes, irreversible brain damage occurs. We'll say it again, because it's so important: to bolster your intelligence you need proper nutrition and plenty of brain stimulation. Now let's see how to get what you need.

MAINTAINING YOUR HEALTH

Since your brain is part of your body, it stands to reason that when the body is not in good shape, the brain cannot be in the best of shape either. Moreover, when you are not well, your brain is diverted from higher-level activities to monitoring your physical condition. Your body functioning slows down to conserve energy and your intellectual processes slow down along with the readjustment in energy level. It's not only smart to be healthy, but you have to be healthy to be smart!

You probably know what you need to keep yourself healthy: the essentials are a balanced diet of wholesome food, exercise, protection from harmful substances, and sufficient rest. While each of these factors is important in total bodily health, there are specific aspects that relate particularly to brain functioning, and we will discuss these shortly. Before we move on to the special needs of your brain, though, look at the checklist that follows. If you cannot answer *yes* to all the items, it is an indication that your health, and therefore your intelligence, is not all that it should be:

	Yes	*No*
1. Are you the right weight for your height and body type?	( )	( )
2. Can you run the length of a block without getting out of breath?	( )	( )
3. Can you touch your toes without bending your knees?	( )	( )
4. Can you take a deep breath and exhale without coughing?	( )	( )
5. Do you wake up feeling refreshed in the morning?	( )	( )
6. Are you free of allergies, headaches, diarrhea, and constipation?	( )	( )
7. Are your hair, skin, and nails in good condition?	( )	( )

If you had to answer *no* to any items, start taking care of yourself right away. Remember, whatever is good for your body is good for your brain and whatever is bad for your body is bad for your brain.

IMPROVING YOUR CIRCULATION

Since your brain gets its nutrients and oxygen through the blood, an efficient circulatory system is essential to a healthy brain. As we pointed out before, just a five-second interruption in the brain's blood supply can cause unconsciousness and permanent cell damage. Conversely, improving the circulatory system of the brain will stimulate it and help put more intelligence at your disposal. This can be accomplished by increasing the blood flow through the arteries that feed the brain, developing the capillaries that branch off to the brain cells, and improving tissue use of oxygen.

To ensure a better flow of blood and oxygen to the brain, you can "train" the carotid arteries, which serve the brain, to open wider. This can be accomplished by any one of three simple methods: underwater swimming, masking, or holding your breath. All these methods involve the same process, namely, momentary increases in the carbon dioxide level in the blood which, paradoxically, increases your oxygen intake. When the carbon dioxide level rises, the valves on the carotid arteries (located in the back of your neck) open wider to let more blood and oxygen flow to the brain. If you induce this condition frequently, after a while the valves open wider permanently. Swimming underwater while holding your breath is the most pleasant way to increase momentarily your CO_2 level and force the carotids to open wider. Each time you swim, go underwater several times, for longer and longer intervals. After a month or two of daily exercise, the carotid valves will be trained to stay open wider. If you do not have access to a pool, another good method is the masking technique developed at the Philadelphia Institute for the Achievement of Human Potential. This method may sound silly, but it works. Simply put a large paper bag over your head and rebreathe your own exhaled air for half a minute. Doing this at half-hour intervals during the day for a period of several weeks will also train the carotid arteries to open wider. You have to be careful in doing this exercise that you use a paper and not a plastic bag, and that you have a small hole in the bag to avoid the possibility of suffocation. Better yet, do this exercise in the presence of another person. If you get the other person to exercise with you, it will keep you from feeling silly and help motivate you both to continue. You can also try just holding your breath for half a minute at frequent intervals during the day. Sit upright, close your eyes, take a deep inhalation through your nose, and hold your breath for a slow count of ten. Exhale slowly and repeat. You can do this exercise for several minutes at a time.

Training the carotid valves to open wider also makes better use of the capillary network feeding the brain cells. Since only those cells near the capillary blood supply are developed, improved flow enables you to keep more cells alive.

Food elements also aid in the development of the brain's circulatory system, notably Vitamin E, Vitamin C, and the B vitamins. Their usefulness and suggested dosages are discussed in the diet section beginning on the following page.

EXERCISES FOR YOUR BRAIN

To keep your brain healthy, you have to give it plenty of exercise. This means providing it with activities that build up and maintain brain cell connections. In a way, this whole book is devoted to that process, focusing on ways to help you use your brain more: to take in more information, to process more information, to think more, to perceive more, to use the emotional aspects of your brain, and to use your long-neglected intuitive abilities. Every time you come across something new, take it in, and integrate it, you establish a new connection and build a framework for increasing your intelligence. Certain parts of your brain that have been getting less use than others are particularly good areas to exercise. These involve the neglected sensory and so-called extrasensory systems (which we discussed in the chapter on hidden powers), and the brain-body coordination systems.

In the chapter "Enhancing Perception," we outlined various exercises for developing your visual perception and increasing your peripheral vision. That chapter also detailed exercises for developing your auditory, olfactory, tactile, and gustatory brain circuits. If you want to keep your brain cells active and connected, it is important that you do those exercises regularly to ensure fuller use of your brain. Another set of exercises involves developing your dexterity and expanding the circuits for brain-body coordination. First of all, there are exercises that involve the integration of perception and fast reactions. This can easily be done in such games as ping-pong and squash. Other exercises for developing coordination involve more delicate tasks. Any activity involving fine movement is good for that purpose and here are a few examples: the game of pick-up sticks, erecting playing-card houses, working on Indian bead designs, playing darts. Another basic dexterity exercise is developing your ability in your less favored hand. If you are right-handed, for example, practice writing, dialing the phone, threading a needle, undoing a knot, and so on, with your left hand. These exercises are not primarily for skill acquisition, but to activate dormant brain circuits.

Most of our physical activity takes place in an upright position, with weight on the feet, so that activities requiring horizontal movements, upside down movements, and hanging suspended by hands are especially helpful. Of these, one of the most difficult exercises to perform, odd as it may sound, is crawling. Try lying flat on your stomach, and propel yourself forward with your hands and your feet! Many of us missed out on the crawling stage in our development, being confined to playpens or put into walkers rather than being allowed to develop the brain circuitry involved in crawling. Win Wenger, in his book *How to Increase Your Intelligence*, emphasizes the importance of crawling in developing the evolutionarily lower regions of the brain, which serve as a foundation for higher intellectual functions. Inverted movements are good for developing your balance and sense of orientation. Hanging upside down on monkey bars is very helpful, as is doing a handstand. Diving also helps. Hanging from your hands and walking via handholds is an excellent all-round exercise that is particularly useful in activating unused brain circuits.

Sleep is also essential to your intelligence. Your brain uses sleep time to consolidate memories of new material learned during the day. Disruption of sleep, on the other hand, disturbs your natural body rhythms and interferes with the ability to concentrate and think productively. Lack of sleep can also cause dream deprivation, which creates mental instability.

BALANCING YOUR DIET

You need a balanced diet not only for your overall health, but for the well-being of your brain. We have become much more aware lately of the importance of proper food to our health and have learned to look for fresh vegetables, fruits, and whole grains, and to limit saturated fats, red meats, and processed food containing additives and preservatives. We are also aware of the dangers of too much sugar, caffeine, and alcohol. Very little attention is given, however, to the effects that various nutrients have on brain functioning. This section provides you with a listing of the vitamins and minerals that are important to a good working brain, along with a description of their role in brain functioning. Your specific need for these nutrients depends on your overall diet and the symptoms you may have. Suggested minimums are given for these dietary supplements, all of which can be purchased at any store that carries vitamins. The dosages suggested vary from the daily minimum requirements formulated by the Food and Drug Administration to much higher dosages. They are based on the consensus among medical experts who have researched the area of mental functioning and its relation to nutrition. Two sources in particular are very helpful if you want to learn about the role of food and the brain in more detail: Michael Lesser's *Nutrition and Vitamin Therapy* and Carl C. Pfeiffer's *Mental and Elemental Nutrients*. The discussion of vitamins and minerals in this section is limited to their usefulness in brain functioning and intelligence. Your overall need for the various nutritional elements listed should be explored separately.

The Vitamins

Vitamins are organic substances found in foods and essential to life, enabling the body to synthesize the special compounds it needs. Each vitamin performs a specific function that cannot be duplicated by any other substance. Although the quantity of vitamins needed is minute, a deficiency can cause serious disruptions to one's health, interfering with the growth, maintenance, and repair of cells. Vitamins work synergistically, interacting with each other, and a lack of one vitamin can also create problems in the body's ability to utilize other vitamins. While vitamins are theoretically present in foods, the amounts contained deviate considerably from the amounts listed in nutritional tables. Vitamins are fragile and easily destroyed by food processing. Eating a so-called balanced diet is, therefore, not necessarily a guarantee that you will obtain the vitamins essential to your health. Further, the minimum daily requirements established by government standards are predicated on keeping you from becoming ill rather than on keeping you maximally healthy. For these reasons, most people need vitamin supplements to keep them functioning at their best.

Vitamin C

This vitamin has many benefits for the brain. Among its most important functions is its ability to work as an antidote to various toxins that you ingest. Vitamin C helps the kidneys excrete such heavy metals as lead and mercury, which have a deleterious effect on the brain. It also helps to reduce stress reactions from bodily or emotional trauma, which ordinarily draw your brain energies away from productive thinking. If taken along with thiamine, Vitamin C helps reduce anxiety. Vitamin C also helps cement the individual cells and has a beneficial effect on capillary development. Foods containing Vitamin C are green peppers and citrus fruit, but these sources usually do not supply a sufficient quantity to deal with the toxins and stresses of our so-called civilized life. The amount of Vitamin C you take should supplement what you lack in your daily diet. Averaging out the 60 mg recommended by the Food and Drug Administration with the 2,300 mg recommended by some researchers, you can conservatively take 500 mg of Vitamin C daily to improve your brain functioning. It is a good idea to take Vitamin C in smaller-sized tablets, say 100 mg at a time, since it is short-lived in the body. Sometimes, you will need to increase your Vitamin C intake. Whenever you are under stress, increase your dosage, again being careful to spread it out in smaller amounts during the day. Also if you smoke a lot or are on a contraceptive pill, you should take more Vitamin C, to help you eliminate the elevated serum copper caused by these two substances. Excess Vitamin C, being water-soluble, is easily eliminated by the body. The possibility of the formation of kidney stones if Vitamin C is taken with calcium supplements is avoided if one takes magnesium as well.

The B Vitamins

The B vitamin family is very important to overall energy and nervous functions. Most diets today are lacking in the B vitamins because they are lost in refining and processing. If you are deficient in any one of the B vitamins, you are usually deficient in the others as well. It is generally a good idea, therefore, to take a B vitamin along with a B-complex tablet or supplement such as wheat germ or brewer's yeast. The body makes better use of the Bs in balance; taking an individual B vitamin in concentrated dosage can cause you to use up the other B vitamins, creating a temporary shortage. You do not have to worry about taking too much of these vitamins, because excess B is easily eliminated by the body. The various B vitamins are described in more detail below.

Vitamin B1 (Thiamine): Thiamine is needed for the general health of the nervous system. A mild lack of B1 causes confusion, fatigue, and irritability, but a severe lack of B1 causes deterioration of manual speed and coordination and a decrement in sensory functioning. If you have any of the symptoms described, try a daily dose of 10 mg to 25 mg of thiamine in a B-complex tablet. If you smoke a lot, drink a lot, or eat a lot of sugar, it is advisable to give yourself an extra boost of B1, since it is depleted by these three conditions. People suffering severe symptoms have been treated with 500 mg twice a day, along with a B complex. You can provide extra B1 in your diet by eating wheat germ and bran, and by using the cooking water from your vegetables.

Vitamin B3 (Niacin): This vitamin is essential to proper brain metabolism. Niacin deficiency causes inability to concentrate and depression. A serious deficiency of B3, in conjunction with a lack of B6, can cause dementia. Mild B3 deficiency can be detected by reddening at the tip of the tongue and enlargement of the taste buds on the tongue's surface, along with white coating at the back of the tongue. If you have a niacin deficiency, start with a dose of 50 mg three times a day after meals. Sometimes people get redness and itchiness with high doses of B3, but this can be counteracted by taking B3 with cold milk. B3 should be taken in conjunction with other B vitamins.

Vitamin B6 (Pyridoxine): A mild deficiency of B6 can create inability to concentrate along with headaches and dizziness. Marked deficiency of B6 can lead to serious mental illness and convulsive symptoms. Physical symptoms of B6 deficiency are dandruff, oily scales around the eyebrows and nose, and numbness and cramping in the arms and legs. The recommended daily minimum for adults is 2 mg but, if it is needed to treat symptoms, up to 1,000 mg may be required. People under stress need higher amounts. Women on birth-control pills who suffer mood changes may be deficient in B6 and require 40 mg daily. Premenstrual blues also suggest a B6 deficiency (take 50 mg to 200 mg). If you have a high-protein diet, your need for B6 will increase. As with the other vitamins in this family, B6 should be balanced by a B complex supplement and, if taken in high doses, by magnesium.

Vitamin B2 (Riboflavin): A lack of B2 causes mental sluggishness. If it occurs in conjunction with a Vitamin A deficiency, it can also affect eyesight. Physical symptoms of B2 deficiency are purple tongue, cracks in the corner of the mouth, chapped-looking lips, and sensitivity to light. As a daily supplement, 10 mg is recommended, but if you are taking doses of the other B vitamins you should increase your B2 intake. B2 produces a bright color in urine, so do not be concerned if this occurs.

Vitamin B12 (Cobalamin): B12 is important for the functioning of all cells, including the brain cells. It participates in the synthesis of RNA and DNA, both important for memory. It helps in transporting oxygen in the blood and it helps combat atrophy of the cerebellum (motor area) of the brain. Deficiency of B12 leads to mental difficulties, including impaired memory and ability to learn and concentrate, and disturbances of perception. B12 deficiency has also been implicated as the cause of many seeming situations of senile dementia. Physical signs of a B12 deficiency include intolerance of noise and light, impairment of the fine movements of the hands and, in severe cases, auditory hallucinations. Although B12 is rarely lacking in the diet, except among vegetarians, a B12 deficiency can be created by the consumption of sugar, which drains the body's vitamin stores. Since B12 is not absorbed well by the intestines, it is best given by injection. Your B12 supplies will probably be sufficient if you eat animal protein, including eggs and dairy products, use brewer's yeast, and avoid sugar. If you take B12, it should be supplemented by folic acid, as described below.

Vitamin B15 (Pangamic Acid): B15 has not been universally recognized as an essential dietary requirement, but it is used widely in some countries. The Russians report it to be helpful in mental retardation, among other conditions. American researchers have found it helpful in stimulating speech in children with delayed speaking ability and in helping autistic children, when given in doses of 50 mg to 100 mg 2 times a day.

Inositol: The need for inositol in humans has not been demonstrated, but its presence in large quantities in all cell tissues, especially the brain, suggests that this nutrient has an important role. Inositol appears to contribute to the transformation of nucleic acids important in forming RNA which is, in turn, important in the storage of memory traces. Inositol has an anti-anxiety effect and has been used instead of Valium. It is particularly effective in cases of insomnia, in anywhere from 500 mg to 1500 mg. Inositol is found naturally in high concentration in lecithin, brewer's yeast, wheat germ, and seed sprouts.

Folic Acid: Folic acid is essential to brain functioning and crucial in the synthesis of RNA and neurotransmitters. A lack of folic acid leads to poor memory as well as general mental sluggishness. Prolonged deficiency may cause mental deterioration. The need for folic acid increases if you are on antibiotics or if you imbibe too much alcohol. Persons on anticonvulsants also have depleted folic acid. Folic acid deficiency is one of the most widespread insufficiencies, and is usually accompanied by a lack of B12. It is particularly seen among the elderly and mentally retarded children, some of whose symptoms may be a result of folic acid deficiency. The recommended dosage of .5 mg for adults per day is rarely met by the average diet, which comes closer to .2 mg a day. People who eat no green or leafy vegetables are particularly lacking in folic acid. The best natural sources are dark green leafy vegetables, such as spinach and parsley, or asparagus and broccoli. Lentils, lima beans, whole grains, and egg yolks also offer fairly high concentrations of folic acid. However, between 50–90 percent of the folic acid in foods may be lost in cooking. Deficiencies of folic acid can be corrected by taking 1 mg of folic acid 2 times a day for 2 to 3 months. Folic acid is sold only in supplements of .4 mg, because it can mask the effects of B12 deficiency. Care must be taken in using folic acid that your B12 level remains adequate.

Choline: Choline is the essential component of acetylcholine, which is a neurotransmitter enabling nerve signals to travel over the synapses. In addition to its role in the transmission of nerve impulses, choline also has been found to be important in aiding memory function. Choline has been recommended in doses of 250 mg as a memory aid. It occurs naturally in granular lecithin (500 mg to a heaping tablespoon) and in brewer's yeast, wheat germ, and soybeans.

Pantothenic Acid: A lack of pantothenic acid leads to fatigue, insomnia, sullenness, and depression. Pantothenic acid is present in nearly all foods and therefore usually sufficiently provided in a balanced diet, but it may be lacking if you eat a lot of processed food. If you are under stress and generally fatigued, you might try 250 mg of pantothenic acid daily—the dosage recommended by the discoverers of this nutrient.

Biotin: Lack of biotin leads to increased sensory sensitivity, especially heightened sensitivity to touch. Deficiencies in biotin also can create depression, drowsiness, and lassitude. The ordinary diet contains sufficient biotin, but this nutrient can be destroyed by eating too many raw egg whites for an extended period of time or being on heavy doses of antiobiotics. Natural sources of biotin are egg yolk, legumes, and nuts.

Vitamin P (Bioflavinoids): The bioflavinoids are important in restoring faulty capillary function and therefore very important to proper circulatory flow in the brain. Rutin, one of the bioflavinoids, also has dual usage as a brain sedative and stimulant. Bioflavinoids are found naturally in the pulp of citrus fruit, but this is lost when juice is strained. They are also found in green peppers, papaya, cantaloupe, and broccoli. Although Vitamin P is not considered an essential part of the daily diet, its usefulness in capillary health suggests you ingest it daily. It has no harmful effects and it prolongs the effectiveness of Vitamin C; 50 mg a day will serve as a brain stimulant, but up to 200 mg a day have been recommended for capillary development.

Vitamin A: Vitamin A is necessary for vision. A deficiency can result in tired, burning, or itchy eyes and inflamed eyelids. Prolonged deficiency can lead to night blindness. Although many plants contain carotene, which the body can convert to usable Vitamin A, especially the yellow and red ones such as apricots, carrots, and beets, the nitrogen in commercial fertilizers that are used for plant growth interferes with the body's ability to use this carotene. Cod liver oil is a good alternate source. Vitamin A can be toxic in large doses, but Michael Lesser reports that adults can take 25,000 units per day indefinitely with safety. In order for the body to utilize Vitamin A, it should be taken in conjunction with Vitamin E and zinc.

Vitamin D: This vitamin is needed for calcium absorption and, therefore, indirectly it can affect the mind by relaxing the nerves and inducing sound sleep. Many diets actually contain too much Vitamin D. Synthetic Vitamin D2 is now added to milk and dairy products and is implicated in the occurrence of abnormal calcium deposits. Natural Vitamin D (D3), which occurs in raw milk, is less likely to cause this condition. Toxicity from Vitamin D can be reduced by using Vitamins C and E.

Vitamin E: Vitamin E aids in the development of the brain's circulatory system. First among its benefits is that it aids in the proliferation of new capillaries and strengthens the walls of blood vessels. Second, Vitamin E is an antioxidant, improving the ability of the brain cells to use the oxygen available. Vitamin E also has a calming effect on the nervous system and helps reduce insomnia.

Although there is considerable controversy in the medical field about the benefits of this vitamin, substantial evidence attests to its importance in circulation. If you are interested, you can find more information on this topic in *Your Heart and Vitamin E* by E. Shute and W. Shute. Vitamin E comes in different forms, and research suggests that they are not all equally helpful. In fact, some of the controversy surrounding the benefits of Vitamin E is based on data collected in studies using less effective forms of this vitamin. For best results get Vitamin E marked *d-alpha tocopherol*. When you begin taking Vitamin E, start off with small doses and build up slowly. Begin with 30 IU daily, doubling the amount to 60 IU after 4 days and to 120 IU after 8 days. Take 120 IU for one week, then increase it to 200 IU for 2 weeks, then double it again to 400 IU and stay on that dosage daily. Take your Vitamin E at the end of your meal. You obtain some Vitamin E in your food, but most diets are very deficient in this substance. It is estimated that the average diet before the advent of processed food contained 170 IU of Vitamin E but that the amount now hovers around 7 IU daily. Foods rich in Vitamin E are wheat germ, leafy green vegetables, and sunflower seeds. Vitamin E has no harmful effects, except when taken in uncontrolled doses by diabetics and persons with high blood pressure.

The Minerals

Minerals, like vitamins, are vital to life and well-being. Unfortunately, less attention is paid to mineral intake than to vitamin intake, even though the body has a lower tolerance for mineral deficiency than for vitamin deficiency. When the level of minerals drops even a small amount, it can jeopardize your physical and mental health.

Even though our bodies are composed of minerals, we cannot manufacture them. We get our minerals from plants which, in turn, get them from the soil, but the minerals in the soil are drained by continuous planting. Commercial fertilizers replenish only three of the minerals depleted by plant cultivation, leaving several important minerals lacking in the soil and therefore in the plants and in our diets.

Calcium
Calcium is important in mediating activity in the entire nervous system. Lack of calcium can result in irritability, tension,

depression, and impairment of memory. Although it is difficult to know when these symptoms are the result of a calcium shortage, it is estimated that 30 percent of the population is calcium-deficient. The average person needs 800 mg daily, but the need increases for persons over fifty, pregnant women, and women on birth control pills. If you are not a milk-drinker (one glass provides 30 percent of the minimum daily requirement) or cheese-eater, you might supplement your diet with calcium tablets of up to 1,000 mg daily. Since calcium interacts with other vitamins and minerals, calcium nutrition must be balanced. Calcium without magnesium can cause calcium deposits. This can be prevented by taking calcium in the form of dolomite, which contains calcium and magnesium. If you take calcium supplements, you need to take zinc supplements as well, since calcium decreases zinc absorption. An excellent source of calcium is eggshell. Although too gritty to eat comfortably, egg shells can be softened in cider vinegar and the calcium made available as calcium acetate.

Magnesium

Magnesium is a tranquilizer for the nervous system and its lack leads to mental fatigue and irritability. Magnesium is plentiful in organically grown green vegetables, but apt to be missing in commercially grown produce, especially that coming from the South. The need for magnesium increases if you drink a lot of alcohol, and many hangover symptoms are also magnesium deficiency symptoms. Birth control pills, too, reduce your magnesium level, as does the onset of menses. The usual American diet provides 300 mg of magnesium daily as compared to 600 mg in the Oriental diet, and it has been suggested that doubling the daily intake would help prevent nervous disorder. Magnesium can be obtained in dolomite tablets, along with calcium. Bathing in Epsom salts (magnesium sulfate) enables you to absorb some magnesium through the skin at the same time that it relaxes you.

Zinc

Zinc plays an important role in helping the body handle toxic heavy metals, which affect general health and brain function. It is also important because of its sedative action on the brain. Zinc deficiency commonly shows up as white spots on the fingernails and may also cause acne, hair loss, and aching joints. The body needs 15 mg a day, but most people get 8–11 mg, and less than a third of one's intake is absorbed. Zinc is deficient in the soil of most growing areas and what is contained in the food tends to be lost in the processing. Alcohol also flushes zinc out of the system. To obtain sufficient daily zinc, supplements of 10 mg each are advisable. If you are very zinc-deficient (with white-spotted nails, for example), between 80 mg to 160 mg daily are recommended.

Selenium

Selenium is important to brain functioning primarily because it protects against the toxic effects of mercury. The suggested daily dose of selenium varies between 50 mcg to 300 mcg, and caution must be used in taking this mineral since it becomes toxic in large quantities (2,000 mcg). Natural sources of selenium include brewer's yeast and garlic.

Manganese

Manganese is important in moderating nervous irritability and in transmitting impulses between nerves and muscles. It helps activate the enzymes that enable the body to use choline and the B vitamins, which are necessary for producing acetylcholine, one of the neurotransmitters. The daily requirement for manganese is 4 mg, this being the amount normally excreted each day. Manganese is largely lost in the processing of food, but whole grains and nuts remain good sources of this mineral.

TOXINS TO THE BRAIN
AND NERVOUS SYSTEM

Protecting your brain against harmful substances is just as important to its functioning as providing it with proper nutrition. Unfortunately, as food has become less nutritious through industrial processing, it has also become more contaminated by pesticides, preservatives, and artificial flavor enhancers. Since the processing removes some of the nutrients that protect us from toxins, we are now even more vulnerable to them. Modern social eating habits also present dangers to our brains and nervous systems. The ubiquitous cocktail party and increased alcohol consumption, for example, are clear hazards to the brain.

Aside from their presence in food, toxins also abound in the air we breathe and water we drink, especially in the form of trace minerals that become damaging to our bodies when present in any concentration. A lot of concern is being expressed these days about the hazards of nuclear testing and radiation, but few people know that recent studies suggest that atomic fallout lowers intellectual activity. States that were subjected to large doses of Strontium 90 from nuclear testing also showed a decrease in the scholastic achievement scores of children exposed to that radiation. While there is not too much you can do to avoid radiation, except to campaign against the wanton use of nuclear power, you can be alert to the other common threats to your brain and avoid them whenever possible.

Toxic Metals

Lead

Lead is an extremely dangerous metal that attacks the nervous system, leading to abnormal brain function, loss of memory and concentration, speech impediments, and mental retardation. Unfortunately, lead is present everywhere in the environment and is easily absorbed by the body. A large percentage is inhaled through auto exhaust fumes and smaller amounts are ingested in food that is contaminated by lead sealants on cans and pesticides. Lead also comes to us courtesy of paint dust, pottery glazes, cigarettes, newsprint, and even some hair dyes. Since the body does not eliminate lead as quickly as it is accumulated, it tends to store in body tissues of animals as well as humans. For this reason, liver, sausages, and organ meats tend to be particularly contaminated and should be avoided.

To avoid airborne lead, the most significant source of lead in our bodies, try to keep yourself away from auto fumes as much as possible. Because lead is a heavy metal, you will inhale more of it the closer you are to street level. It may be difficult to change your place of residence, but when you travel, ask for a hotel room on an upper floor and avoid bedrooms that face a heavily trafficked street. If you grow vegetables, plant them away from roads and if you buy vegetables from farms, avoid those adjacent to a highway, where produce is apt to be lead-contaminated. Avoid jogging or biking on a busy street and do your exercising in hours when traffic is at a minimum.

To protect yourself against the lead which you do absorb, one of the best antidotes is Vitamin C in dosages recommended in the vitamin section. Also, if your body has sufficient calcium and zinc, you will absorb less lead and suffer less toxicity.

Mercury

Mercury accumulates in the brain and, if concentrated enough, damages neural elements, leading eventually to derangement. It has been recently suspected that many of the signs of senility may actually be the consequence of mercury accumulation. Most of the mercury we are exposed to comes from food. Fish becomes contaminated with mercury discharged into rivers and lakes by industry, and the amount of mercury poisoning is directly proportional to the size of the fish. For this reason big fish, such as tuna and swordfish, should be at the bottom of your list. Also avoid patent medicines containing calomel, found in some laxatives, which contains mercury. Since there is not much that can be done to treat mercury poisoning, avoid it as much as possible.

Aluminum

The inhalation or ingestion of aluminum appears to produce brain damage and there is evidence that aluminum may be partially responsible for senile dementia. The biggest source of aluminum pollution is cookware, and the easiest way to avoid aluminum poisoning is to avoid cooking with it, including the use of aluminum foil. Be particularly wary of cooking acid fruits in aluminum ware. Other sources of aluminum are table salt, deodorants, some toothpastes, and baking powder. If you cannot find a commercial baking powder without aluminum, you can make your own with the following recipe: two parts cream of tartar, one part baking soda, and one part cornstarch.

Cadmium

Cadmium can lead to intoxication of the brain, hyperactivity, and impaired verbal abilities. In nature it exists in balance with zinc and is often found in items made from impure zinc. Living downwind from a zinc smelting plant can expose you to cadmium as can cigarette smoke and burning coal. The best antidote to cadmium is zinc. If you have sufficient zinc in your system, you will absorb less cadmium.

Copper

Copper is a necessary trace mineral, but it becomes toxic in excess. Since copper is abundant in the diet, you are much more likely to have too much copper than too little. In excessive amounts, copper can cause learning difficulties, stuttering, and even autism. In addition to its presence in food, copper is ordinarily obtained from water, copper plumbing, and copper cookware. If you take the daily minimum requirement of zinc and manganese, you will keep your copper level in proper balance.

Bismuth

Excess bismuth can lead to difficulties in memory, estimating time and distance, and to disturbances in vision, hearing, and speech. Bismuth is contained in over-the-counter remedies for stomach upset and diarrhea. Check the labels on these products and avoid repeated use.

Bromine

Excess bromine can cause poor memory and mental dullness. Bromine salts are contained in products for acid indigestion and excessive use should be avoided.

Other Harmful Substances

Monosodium Glutamate

MSG is widely used in prepared food as a flavor enhancer and may cause brain damage, especially in infants. It is the agent responsible for the dizziness known to some diners as the *Chinese-restaurant syndrome*. Check labels of prepared food for MSG, and ask your favorite Chinese restaurant to leave it out of your dinner. Commercial flavor enhancers like Accent are basically MSG.

Aspartame

This is a new sugar substitute that may cause the same kind of brain damage as MSG. Stay on the safe side and avoid it.

Carbon Monoxide

Carbon monoxide gets into your system primarily from auto exhaust. It is a threat to your intelligence because it prevents the blood from carrying oxygen to your brain. While doing strenuous exercises, your carbon monoxide intake will be increased if you are exposed to auto exhaust, so avoid jogging in traffic. Eating lunch at a sidewalk café, though pleasant, also exposes you to increased carbon monoxide.

The Common Sins

Alcohol

One of the most dangerous threats to your brain is alcohol. Too much liquor can literally wipe out your brain cells. One drinking bout can cost you the loss of millions of brain cells. If you want to increase your intelligence and maintain it into old age, avoid drinking too much at one time. A daily cocktail, or glass of wine, or a couple of beers appear to aid longevity, but please note the "or" in that statement!

Tobacco

We are all aware of the harmful effects of smoking on the lungs and the heart, but smoking also has a harmful effect on the brain, leading to an increase in beta waves and a decrease in alpha-wave activity. Translated into other terms, heavy smoking can impede your creative brain activity. Large doses of nicotine can also produce tremors.

Refined Sugar

If you have a sweet tooth, that is bad for your brain as well as your teeth. Overuse of refined sugar burns up the B vitamins in your body and exposes you to the dangers of B deficiency: mental sluggishness, poor concentration, poor memory, impaired synthesis of neurotransmitters, among others. Excess sugar can also create functional hypoglycemia (sugar starvation), which leads to a loss of memory, decreased concentration, and confusion. If you can't resist sweets, balance sugar in your diet with B supplements.

SUGGESTED READING

INTELLIGENCE:
WHAT IT IS AND HOW IT GROWS

Blum, Jeffrey. *Pseudoscience and Mental Ability*. New York: Monthly Review Press, 1978.

Engelmann, Siegfried and Therese. *Give Your Child a Superior Mind*. New York: Simon & Schuster, Inc., 1966.

Ferguson, Marilyn. *The Brain Revolution*. New York: Taplinger Publishing Co., Inc., 1973.

Gould, Steven Jay. *The Mismeasure of Man*. New York: W. W. Norton & Co., Inc., 1981.

Kamin, Leon J. *The Science and Politics of IQ*. Potomac, Md.: Lawrence Erlbaum Associates, Inc., 1974.

Montessori, Maria. *The Absorbent Mind* (1949) (C. A. Claremont, trans.). New York: Holt, Rinehart & Winston, 1967.

Restak, Richard M. *The Brain: The Last Frontier*. Garden City, N.Y.: Doubleday & Co., Inc., 1979.

Sternberg, Robert J. "Who's Intelligent," *Psychology Today*, April, 1982, Vol. 16, No. 4, pp. 30–39.

Whimbey, Arthur, with Linda Shaw Whimbey. *Intelligence Can Be Taught*. New York: E. P. Dutton, 1975.

PROCESSING VERBAL INFORMATION

Buzan, Tony. *Use Both Sides of Your Brain*. New York: E. P. Dutton, 1977.

Festinger, Leon. *A Theory of Cognitive Dissonance*. Palo Alto, Ca.: Stanford University Press, 1957.

Maberly, Norman C. *Mastering Speed Reading*. New York: Signet Book, The New American Library, Inc., 1966.

Schick, G. B., and M. M. May. *Reading: Process and Pedagogy*. Milwaukee, Wis.: National Reading Conference, 1970.

Wason, P. C. and P. N. Johnson-Laird. *Psychology of Reasoning.* Cambridge, Mass.: Harvard University Press, 1972.

ENHANCING PERCEPTION

Dodwell, P. C. *Visual Pattern Recognition.* New York: Holt, Rinehart & Winston, 1970.

Gregory, R. L. *Eye and Brain*, Third Edition. New York: McGraw-Hill Paperbacks, 1978.

IMPROVING MEMORY

Cermak, Laird S. *Improving Your Memory.* New York: McGraw-Hill Paperbacks, 1976.

Loftus, Elizabeth. *Memory.* Reading, Mass.: Addison-Wesley Publishing Co., Inc., 1980.

Lorayne, Harry and Jerry Lucas. *The Memory Book.* New York: Ballantine Books, Inc., 1974.

Luria, A. R. *The Mind of Mnemonist.* New York: Basic Books, Inc., 1968.

Ostrander, Sheila and Lynn Schroeder, with Nancy Ostrander. *Superlearning.* New York: Delacorte Press, 1979.

MODES OF THINKING

Bruner, J. S., R. R. Oliver, P. M. Greenfield, et. al. *Studies in Cognitive Growth.* New York: John Wiley & Sons, Inc., 1966.

de Bono, Edward. *Lateral Thinking.* New York: Harper & Row Publishers, Inc., 1970.

Engel, S. Morris. *With Good Reason: An Introduction to Informal Fallacies.* New York: St. Martin's Press, Inc., 1976.

Gordon, William J. J. *Synectics.* New York: Collier Books, MacMillan Publishing Co., Inc., 1961.

Luria, A. R. *Cognitive Development: Its Cultural and Social Foundations.* Cambridge, Mass.: Harvard University Press, 1978.

McKim, Robert. *Experiences in Visual Thinking.* Monterey, Ca.: Brooks/Cole Publishing Company, 1972.

Mayer, R. E. *Thinking and Problem Solving.* Glenview, Ill.: Scott, Foresman & Company, 1977.

Osborn, Alex F. *Applied Imagination.* New York: The Scribner Book Companies, Inc., 1963.

Perkins, D. N. *The Mind's Best Work.* Cambridge, Mass.: Harvard University Press, 1981.

Radford, John and Andrew Burton. *Thinking: Its Nature and Development.* London: John Wiley & Sons, Inc., 1974.

Revlin, Russell and Richard E. Mayer. *Human Reasoning.* New York: John Wiley & Sons, Inc., 1978.

Sommer, Robert. *The Mind's Eye.* New York: Delacorte Press, 1978.

Wallas, G. *The Art of Thought.* New York: Harcourt, 1926.

Whimbey, Arthur and Jack Lockhead. *Problem Solving and Comprehension.* Philadelphia, Pa.: The Franklin Institute Press, 1979.

THE POWER OF NEGATIVE THINKING

Luchins, A. S. "Mechanization in Problem Solving," *Psychological Monographs,* 1942, 54 (Whole No. 48).

Postman, Neil and Charles Weingartner. *Teaching as a Subversive Activity.* New York: Dell Publishing Co., Inc., 1969.

Rockeach, Milton. *The Open and Closed Mind.* New York: Basic Books, 1960.

RAISING YOUR IQ

Block, N. J. and Gerald Dworkin (eds.). *The IQ Controversy.* New York: Pantheon Books, 1976.

Feder, Bernard. *The Complete Guide to Taking Tests.* Englewood Cliffs, N.J.: Prentice-Hall, Inc., 1979.

Jacobs, Paul. *Up the IQ*. New York: Wyden Books, 1977.

Jensen, Arthur R. "How Much Can We Boost IQ and Scholastic Achievement?" *Harvard Educational Review*, 1969, 33, pp. 1–123.

Strenio, Jr., Andrew J. *The Testing Trap*. New York: Rawson, Wade Publishers, Inc., 1981.

EMOTIONS AND INTELLIGENCE

Benson, Herbert. *The Relaxation Response*. New York: William Morrow & Co., Inc., 1975.

Davitz, J. R. *The Language of Emotion*. New York: Academic Press, Inc., 1969.

Halstead, W. C. *Brain and Intelligence*. Chicago: University of Chicago Press, 1974.

McClelland, David D. *The Achievement Motive*. New York: Appleton-Century-Crofts, 1953.

HIDDEN POWERS OF THE MIND

Boss, Medard. *The Analysis of Dreams*. New York: Philosophical Library, Inc., 1958.

Brown, Barbara B. *New Mind, New Body*. New York: Harper & Row, Publishers, Inc., 1974.

Butler, W. E. *How to Read the Aura, Practice Psychometry, Telepathy and Clairvoyance*. New York: Warner Destiny Books, 1978.

Ebon, Martin (ed.). *The Signet Handbook of Parapsychology*. New York: Signet Book, The New American Library, Inc., 1978.

Koestler, Arthur. *The Roots of Coincidence*. New York: Vintage Books, 1973.

LeShan, Lawrence. *Alternate Realities*. New York: M. Evans & Co., Inc., 1976.

Ornstein, Robert E. *The Psychology of Consciousness*. San Francisco: W. H. Freeman & Company, 1972.

Ostrander, S. and L. Schroeder. *Psychic Discoveries Behind the Iron Curtain*. New York: Bantam Books, Inc., 1971.

Panati, Charles. *Supersenses*. New York: Quadrangle/The New York Times Book Co., 1974.

Van Over, Raymond. *Total Meditation*. Collier Books, Macmillan Publishing Co., Inc., 1978.

Wittrock, M. C. (ed.). *The Human Brain*. Englewood Cliffs, N.J.: Prentice-Hall, Inc., 1977.

THE CARE AND FEEDING
OF THE BRAIN

Lesser, Michael. *Nutrition and Vitamin Therapy*. New York: Grove Press, Inc., 1980.

Pfeiffer, Carl C. *Mental and Elemental Nutrients*. New Canaan, Conn.: Keats Publishing, Inc., 1975.

Rose, Steven. *The Conscious Brain*. New York: Alfred A. Knopf, Inc., 1975.

Scientific American, September 1979, Vol. 241, Whole Number 3.

Shute, E. and W. Shute. *Your Heart and Vitamin E*. Detroit: The Cardiac Society, 1956.

Wenger, Win. *How to Increase Your Intelligence*. New York: A Dell Book, Dell Publishing Co., Inc., 1975.

INDEX